£7·95

Child abuse and its consequences
Observational approaches

RACHEL CALAM

Department of Clinical Psychology, Royal Manchester Children's Hospital, Pendelbury

CRISTINA FRANCHI

Social Services Department, London Borough of Waltham Forest

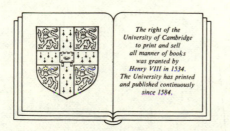

The right of the
University of Cambridge
to print and sell
all manner of books
was granted by
Henry VIII in 1534.
The University has printed
and published continuously
since 1584.

CAMBRIDGE UNIVERSITY PRESS

Cambridge
New York   New Rochelle   Melbourne   Sydney

Published by the Press Syndicate of the University of Cambridge
The Pitt Building, Trumpington Street, Cambridge CB2 1RP
32 East 57th Street, New York, NY 10022, USA
10 Stamford Road, Oakleigh, Melbourne 3166, Australia

First published 1987

Printed in Great Britain at
the University Press, Cambridge

British Library cataloguing in publication data
Calam, Rachel
Child abuse and its consequences:
observational approaches.
1. Child abuse–Services–Great Britain
I. Title II. Franchi, Cristina
362.7'044   HV751.A6

Library of Congress cataloguing in publication data
Calam, Rachel.
Child abuse and its consequences.
Bibliography
Includes index.
1. Child abuse. 2. Interviewing in child abuse.
3. Behavior assessment in children. 4. Abused children.
I. Franchi, Cristina. II. Title.
HV6626.5.C35   1987   362.7'044   86–21535

ISBN 30277 3 hard covers
ISBN 31614 6 paperback

SE

TO HUGH AND PETER

Contents

Names and other specific details that might serve to identify individuals, families or the location of the main body of the research have been changed in order to preserve anonymity. The views expressed in the book are the authors' own and are not meant to represent NSPCC or any other policy.

Acknowledgements

This book owes a great deal to the children, the mothers and the staff at the Family Centre and NSPCC Special Units where the research was carried out, and we hope that it will be of use to them, and to those who follow them. We would like to thank everyone who participated in the research or who helped to make it possible. We would like to thank the nursery staff for allowing us to work so closely with them in the Family Centre. We thank them, too, for the many hours that we have spent in discussion of the children and families, and of associated issues. In particular, the Matron supplied a great deal of the information that we have included on the children's development, and much of the follow-up information was provided by her. We would also like to thank Brian Roycroft and all the people in the Community Health and Education Departments who helped to make the Newcastle follow-up possible.

We are grateful to Cliff Davies for providing the initial contact with the Family Centre, for working with us in planning and discussing the study, and for the energy and support that he provided in obtaining funding for the second phase of the research. His help has contributed a great deal to the observational work. Brian Clark gave generously of his time in setting up the computer analysis of the observational data. We also gratefully acknowledge the financial support of the then Social Science Research Council for parts of this work.

Many people have helped us in the preparation of the manuscript. We gratefully acknowledge the assistance of Glynn Owens in planning Chapter 12, and his comments on this part of the manuscript. We are also grateful to David Pilgrim for his comments on parts of the text. In particular, we would like to thank Peter Elliott for his patience in reading an earlier draft of the complete manuscript; his careful reading and thoughtful comments have added a great deal to the quality of the book.

Lastly, we thank Ida and Francesca Franchi, Peter Argall and Hugh Wagner for their encouragement, support, and practical help throughout the research period and the preparation of the manuscript.

1   *Introduction*

The young child which lieth in the cradle is both wayward and full of affections; and though his body be but small, yet he hath a reat [wrong-doing] heart, and is altogether inclined to evil . . . If this sparkle be suffered to increase, it will rage over and burn down the whole house.
Robert Cleaver and John Dod (1621) *A Godly Form of Household Government*
(Cited in de Mause, 1974, p. 316)

In the night they do wake up and they get a smack – well they don't get a smack actually, they get put in my bed . . . he's a little bleeder, but I love that in a child. It keeps you going.
Connie, mother of a seriously injured child, 1982

RECOGNITION OF THE PROBLEM

The cruel treatment of children has a very long history; the history of concern over child abuse is comparatively short. In ancient times children were used for ritual sacrifice, and unwanted children, particularly girls, were exposed on hillsides and left to die (de Mause, 1974). In more recent times the Industrial Revolution saw very young children working long hours, tending machines in mills and factories, scrambling up chimneys and crawling down mines. The dreadful injuries suffered by many of these children, as well as the large numbers of children living as best they could on the streets of major cities, drew the attention of such figures as Shaftesbury and Barnardo who were to spearhead the great reform movements of the nineteenth century. The harsh usage of these children reflects the low value placed on the lives and happiness of disadvantaged children in comparatively recent times.

It was only when general social conditions began to improve that interest slowly came to focus on the abuse of children by their parents. As Kempe (1979) has commented, it is only in societies where causes of child death such as disease and malnutrition are under control and child mortality is expected to be low that child abuse can become an issue. Foucault (1976) also suggests that the concern for improved standards of care of children in the eighteenth century arose from a need to raise the general health of the population for industrial and political purposes. Physical abuse of children in the form of

1

what we now know as non-accidental injury (NAI) was to come to the public eye through well-publicised cases such as that of Mary Ellen in 1874. The National Society for the Prevention of Cruelty to Children (NSPCC) was founded in 1884, following on from the establishment of the Royal Society for the Prevention of Cruelty to Animals, who provided premises for some of the early child abuse work. Lynch (1985) provides an excellent history of child abuse up to 1962 (see also Jones, 1982; Radbill, 1968).

The rights of parents to treat their children as they wished had, up to 1889, been enshrined in law, but the Prevention of Cruelty Act, passed in that year, secured the protection of children suffering the extremes of cruel treatment. The responsibility for the care of such children rested with non-medical personnel, whose concern was for the quality of life experienced by the child. This care had now become the responsibility of state and charity-funded professionals such as social workers.

Initially, there was little medical involvement. In the 1940s, however, the radiographer Caffey identified a 'syndrome' which included long bone fractures and subdural haematoma seen on the X-rays of children (Caffey, 1946), and in 1962 the paediatrician Henry Kempe and his co-workers described the 'Battered Child Syndrome', later to be referred to as the 'Battered Baby Syndrome' (Kempe *et al.*, 1962). Once medical criteria were available for diagnosis, early detection became the responsibility of the medical establishment, who could identify cases as they came into casualty. This established a new role for medical practitioners.

In Britain, the death of Maria Colwell in 1973 coincided with an initiative headed by Sir Keith Joseph to look at the 'cycle of deprivation' across generations. This coincidence gave tremendous impetus to the establishment of a new role for the NSPCC in the development of better ways of understanding and working with this problem, and the 1970s saw a major expansion in research and facilities aimed at the prevention of physical abuse of children. Kempe sees the development of the recognition of child abuse as a problem as passing through the stages of denial, attention to the most lurid features, and then attention to more subtle forms (see Smith, 1984).

THE DEVELOPMENT OF DEFINITIONS

Parton (1979) gives a detailed account of a four-stage process by which child abuse came to be recognised and defined. The four stages are: (1) the discovery of the problem, through the use of X-ray; (2) its diffusion as a problem, through the publicity afforded the case of Maria Colwell; (3) the consolidation of the problem, with the state and NSPCC taking responsibility; and finally (4) the stage of reification, with the problem being accepted as a 'natural phenomenon' that should automatically receive professional attention.

Three approaches to the management of child abuse cases are identified by

Parton: (1) the penal, with emphasis on justice for the injured party and punishment of the offender; (2) the medical, which sees deviance as a result of external forces requiring prevention and cure; and (3) the social welfare model, which can be divided into (i) the traditional, compassionate rehabilitation view which sees the parents as psychologically or emotionally inadequate and in need of therapy, and (ii) the radical view which sees a need for social reorganisation, and has social processes and social change as its focus.

The medical model, which was particularly influential at the beginning of this recent expansion of interest in the problem, carried with it a number of tacit assumptions: that child abuse was a recognisable and deviant form of behaviour; and, given that it was a recognised syndrome, that a cure was possible and prevention a state to be aimed at. Since no one in their right mind would damage a young child, mental imbalance was implicit. The groundwork for this disease model had already been laid by the Infanticide Act 1938 which acknowledged that mothers might kill their children soon after birth if in a state of emotional disturbance, and the image of the 'child abuser' as a particular category of abnormal individual was easy to establish.

This model led to a considerable literature on the 'characteristics' of abusing parents, which was the first area to receive systematic study. With cases identified or reified by medical workers, and then handed on to the traditional social welfare school, the model adopted assumed an underlying psychopathology within the parents which could be uncovered through the study of parents who had injured their children. The implication for therapy was that although the child was the recognised victim in need of protection, it was through studying and helping parents that change could be brought about. The consequence of this model was that termination of physically injurious behaviour towards the child together with some degree of attitudinal change away from the pathological on the behalf of the parent tended to be seen as an adequate aim of and end-point to therapy.

At the same time, the 1960s had seen the accumulated impact of extremely influential work by Bowlby (1953), who argued that bonding between mother and infant was essential to the mental health of the developing individual. Bowlby argued on the one hand that the rich environment provided by a good mother–child relationship was the optimal setting for healthy mental development, and on the other hand that the disruption of this bond, or 'maternal deprivation', would be likely to have dire consequences for the child. As evidence for the latter, he cited studies of children reared in institutions who had suffered mental retardation. Further, he stated:

It must never be forgotten that even a bad parent who neglects her child is none-the-less providing much for him. Except in the worst instances, she is giving him food and shelter, comforting him in distress, teaching him simple skills, and above all is providing him with that continuity of human care on which his sense of security rests. He may be ill-fed and ill-sheltered, he may be very dirty and suffering from disease, but, unless his parents have wholly rejected him, he is secure in the knowledge that there is someone to whom he is of value . . . it is against this background that the reason why children thrive better in bad homes than in good institutions, and why children with bad parents are apparently unreasonably, so attached to them, can be understood.

(p. 78)

There were problems with Bowlby's arguments which were not fully appreciated at the time. Bowlby was taken as stating that maternal care was the best of all available alternatives unless the child had been 'wholly rejected', but determining when such a point has been reached is far from easy. Many of Bowlby's comments were based on poorer standards of institutional care than those currently available. Also, it could not be assumed that continuity of care ensured a sense of security in the child. On the other hand, Bowlby was well aware that leaving the familial home for alternative care might be the start of a series of institutional or foster experiences which would involve a greater degree of damage than that caused by conditions at home. At intervals in his writing he suggested that a 'mother substitute' could be an adequate alternative to the natural mother, a fact which tended to be ignored as his theories were woven into child care practice.

These lines of argument and the concept of parental psychopathology, combined with the notion of bonding and the undesirability of substitute care, contributed to the search for characteristics of abusing parents, and ways of helping them to care for their children in the community. It was acknowledged that abuse was likely to have an effect on the child, and characteristics of abused children were also sought, although long-term studies of such children continue to be rare. As the work on characterisation of abusing parents and abused children has been influential in determining the approach to provision of help for families where abuse is known to have occurred, and in directing research in this area, we summarise some of the main findings below.

CHARACTERISTICS OF THE ABUSING PARENT

Research suggests that abusing parents do not provide the sort of emotional environment that would foster normal development. Steele & Pollock (1968) found abusing parents had unrealistically high expectations of their children from a young age and expected them to respond with love in a non-age-appropriate way (see also Baher *et al.*, 1976). A mother in their study commented:

I have never felt loved in all my life. When the baby was born, I thought he would love me, but when he cried all the time, it meant he didn't love me, so I hit him.

Abusing parents see the child in terms of their own emotional needs, not as a separate entity with needs of his or her own. High expectations of the child are coupled with little knowledge of age-appropriate or development-appropiate behaviours (Steele & Pollock, 1968; Martin & Rodeheffer, 1976). What is considered desirable behaviour at one stage of development irrespective of its appropriateness, might later be seen as undesirable by the mother. Such maternal behaviour is aptly described in a quote from Tennes in Kempe & Kempe (1978):

Keith was seven months old and beginning to have activity which was increasingly irritating to his mother. Activity during nappy changing she found most unbearable and she said 'I had to whack him again and again to make him hold still.' Keith was observed while being changed, lying completely immobile, intently watching his mother's hands with a serious expression on his face. Three months later she complained that Keith had learned his lesson only too well. During changing and dressing he now became quite limp, failing to hold his hand to have his shirt put on. Mother said she would '. . . have to show him he could only go so far before he got the flat of her hand again.'   (p. 31)

Martin & Rodeheffer (1976) have commented that unrealistic and distorted expectations are the hallmark of most abusing parents. Crying, dirtying nappies or clothes, or breaking a toy can all be seen as deliberately naughty behaviour by the parents. They might have a rigid set of rules to which the child is expected to adhere irrespective of his or her age, needs or capabilities (Steele & Pollock, 1968). They can be inconsistent disciplinarians, making it difficult for the child to understand the sudden harsh punishments that are meted out (Parke & Collmer, 1975; Gelles, 1980).

Spinetta & Rigler (1980) reviewed the literature on abusing parents and concluded that:

1.   The abusing parent(s) has a history of a deprived childhood and/or of abuse.
2.   The abusing parent brings to his or her role mistaken notions of child rearing.
3.   The abusing parent has 'a general defect in character structure allowing aggressive impulses to be expressed too freely'.
4.   Socio-economic factors may place additional stresses on the parent but these stresses are not in themselves sufficient to cause abuse.

Kempe & Kempe (1978) reached similar conclusions and made the additional point that the abusing parents view the child as unlovable or disappointing. This emphasises the interactional nature of the abuse and offers a possible explanation for why not all children in an abusive family are necessarily abused or abused to the same extent. Although not all abused children become abusing parents (Zigler, 1980), abusing parents do appear to have been victims of deprivation and abuse themselves. Kempe & Kempe (1978) suggest that the nature of the parents' own childhood experiences limits their ability to choose between parenting models, so that they repeat the parenting pattern to which they were exposed; one might see in this process the transmission between generations of the 'cycle of deprivation' (critically reviewed by Rutter & Madge, 1976).

CHARACTERISTICS OF ABUSED CHILDREN

Martin & Beezley (1977) developed a list of nine characteristics that they had observed in a group of 50 abused children. These characteristics have often been quoted subsequently, and are as follows:

1.   Impaired capacity to enjoy life
2.   Psychiatric symptoms, e.g. enuresis, tantrums, hyperactivity, bizarre behaviour
3.   Low self-esteem
4.   School learning problems
5.   Withdrawal
6.   Opposition
7.   Hypervigilance
8.   Compulsivity
9.   Pseudo-mature behaviour

They commented that several maxims could be drawn out from their research. Of particular importance was the observation, made by many researchers, that there is no one personality profile of 'the abused child', and each child will respond differently to his or her individual circumstances. They noted that the complete environment, including rejection and changes of caretaker, periods of fostering and so on, was likely to have a greater impact on the child's development than the act of physical abuse itself. Further, they observed that any personality trait the child exhibited that appeared to be a product of the abusive environment should be viewed from different perspectives. On the one hand, a particular trait might appear to be a developmental delay; on the other, it might be seen as a necessary adaptation to an abusive environment. The chameleon-like adaptability to different environments of the children in this study was noted, which again is a survival mechanism.

Let us look at some of these characteristics of abused children in more detail. Martin & Beezley describe pseudo-mature behaviour thus:

. . . The compulsive and pseudo-adult children were locked into styles which are not conducive to age appropriate enjoyment or flexibility. The pseudo-adult child has forfeited his right to feel and act like a child, instead planning his life for the pleasure of adults rather than for himself.

Such descriptions hint at what might be the psychological consequences developmentally of the experiences of being abused. Abused children must concentrate on keeping their parents happy and avoiding harm and consequently may miss out on play and make-believe, not feeling confident to explore their environment freely. Beezley, Martin & Kempe (1976) have described how abused children in therapy found it difficult to 'let go' and tried to find out what they were *expected* to do with the toys – in other words, they were playing to please the therapist. They had low self-esteem, seeing themselves as stupid or naughty and underestimating themselves, saying they could not do things that were clearly within their ability. Such underestimation might be another adaptive response: it might be safer not to attempt something rather than attempt it and risk failure and possibly punishment (Martin & Rodeheffer, 1976). This response might also be carried over into the school situation later.

Some abused children show extreme attentiveness – what Ounsted has called 'frozen watchfulness' (Kempe & Kempe, 1978). They stare continually, constantly scanning the environment, avoiding eye contact and keeping their faces immobile. They are fearful and shy and have not learnt to please with smiling, social behaviour. Although they may avoid punishment by such behaviour, optimal conditions for learning through exploration of parents, toys and environment are also missing. In addition, these children are extraordinarily passive and accepting of whatever happens to them. They will submit to excruciatingly painful treatment in hospital with barely a whimper (personal communication, Family Centre Matron).

However, abused children do not fall into a homogenous group: some are compliant and anxious to please, others manifest 'demon' symptoms, yet others switch from sweet, compliant behaviour to disruptive behaviour without apparent provocation. Kempe & Kempe (1978) have estimated that at least a quarter of young abused children exhibit what they have christened 'demon' symptoms. Such children are difficult to manage, not listening to directions and seemingly impervious to disapproval. They move constantly and cannot play with other children, continually hitting out at them. Their language is as aggressive as their behaviour. Some of these children have been thought to be suffering from neurologically determined hyperactivity, but Kempe & Kempe suggest that their behaviour is more probably a manifestation of disorganised anxiety. They have come to view aggression as their only outlet and have learnt a negative mode of coping with their situation.

Whichever of these patterns of behaviour an abused child adopts, none would seem to facilitate learning or the verbalisation of feelings and intentions. It is not surprising, therefore, that there is evidence of delayed language development in abused children, particularly as regards the expressive mode. Elmer (1977a) observed that abused children used less expressive language and Blager & Martin (1976) suggested that in their study the children were not using language as a vehicle for ideas but rather as another means of avoiding punishment, trying both to evade further questioning and to ingratiate themselves with the experimenter. Some children appeared highly solicitous, showing sympathy for the experimenter, and Malone (1966) has suggested they might use such behaviour in an attempt to appease their parents. Abused children often find it difficult to express their feelings, and in addition Kempe & Kempe (1978) found they avoided talking about their family or life outside the playroom.

The work discussed so far has described the behaviours of abused children and suggested that some of these behaviours might be interpreted as adaptations to the environment in which the child finds him- or herself. There have been some attempts to consider the long-term prognosis for the child. Martin *et al.* (1974), reviewing the existing literature on the development of abused children, concluded that they are at high risk for damage to the central nervous system and maldevelopment of ego function. There is, however, conflicting evidence on the extent to which physical or developmental deviations antedate abuse, either through being of a congenital nature or being the result of rearing in an abusive or deprived environment. Kempe & Kempe (1978) state that there is usually early evidence, by the end of the first year of life, of a 'deviance' in development in abused children, with delays in motor, social and cognitive development. They conclude:

. . . it is our impression, as yet unproven, that much of the retardation observed in abused children is related less to the physical abuse itself than to the neglect and emotional abuse that most often accompany it.   (p. 45)

Whatever the genesis of these developmental deviations, they have certainly been detected by their teachers in school-aged abused children, in studies that have used the Bristol Social Adjustment Guide (BSAG) questionnaire. Roberts, Lynch & Duff (1978) in a follow-up of their sample found a quarter of the children who remained with their natural parents were considered maladjusted by their teachers, most often being characterised on the BSAG as over-aggressive.

The longer-term effects of abuse on the child's psychological development are considered in more detail in Chapter 2, where a long-term follow-up study of the school adjustment of children abused 5 – 10 years previously is reported.

Some studies have looked at the contribution that the child may make to abuse by the parents. Kadushin & Martin (1981) discussed the way in which the child might provoke an attack. Another study, by Bender (1976), found that some abused children might 'play the victim' and invite harm, a behavioural pattern that carried over into foster homes where the children were re-injured.

PHYSICAL CHASTISEMENT AND PHYSICAL ABUSE

Gil (1970) sets child abuse in the context of a society that tolerates physical chastisement of children. He puts forward the view that physical abuse is facilitated by tolerance of physical force as a means of control. It is suggested that all children, particularly those subject to regimes of discipline involving physical chastisement, are at potential risk of abuse. Rather than seeking a specific pathology in the parent, such a perspective sees abuse as an extreme of a continuum which includes the entire range of disciplinary practices. Gil found that more than half the cases of physical injury that he studied in a large survey involved an act of physical chastisement that had gone too far.

Newson & Newson (1963, 1968, 1976) in a longitudinal study of attitudes to child rearing in industrial England in the 1960s found considerable variation in the opinions of parents regarding physical chastisement of children, and a general tolerance of physical discipline as a means of control. In interviews, 62% of the parents of 1-year-old children said that they regularly used smacking as a form of discipline. At 4 years of age, 75% of the children were being smacked once a week or more, compared with 41% at 7 years. A small group of parents appeared particularly committed to physical control: 8% of the parents of 7-year-olds were smacking once a day or more. Some parents reported the regular use of an implement, such as a belt or hairbrush. These families could be seen as bordering on physical abuse of their children; to some, their behaviour would already be viewed as such. Physical abuse could then be seen as part of a continuum of child rearing practice.

In line with the continuum model, Zigler (1983) suggests that the two-category system of classification of parents into those who physically abuse their children and those who do not should be replaced by a continuum that has affection at one end and murder at the other, with occasional violence to children in between. He suggests that this would enable professionals to deal with acts that do not fit present legal or medical definitions of abuse. For a full discussion of these issues see Zigler (1980, 1983).

THE PROBLEM OF DEFINITION

As Zigler points out, the significance of the type of definition of child abuse used should not be minimised. As the rest of this book will show, physical injury *per se* is not a sufficient criterion on which to base decisions about the quality of parental care, yet most intervention with families has to use this as a means of gaining cooperation, or control.

Zigler (1983) suggests a series of levels of definition which might make the task of helping and studying families rather easier. Each level carries with it different administrative, procedural and research implications. The first three categories of definition correspond to some extent to the different professional perspectives discussed by Parton (1979).

1.   *Medical.* A very stringent form of definition. Symptoms are seen in terms of nature and severity, of acute or chronic status.
2.   *Legal.* A similarly stringent form of definition, allowing intervention in family life if certain explicit standards are violated, and there is

supporting documentary evidence. The family can be subjected to
varying degrees of coercion.
3.   *Sociological.* This definition allows for the inclusion of more diffuse
concepts. Definition is a task of judgement in relation to concepts of
acceptable or unacceptable parenting practices. The correction of the
family's ecology in terms of political, social and human values is
sought.
4.   *Research.* The definitions used here need to encompass all of the
above, in order to study and develop programmes for prevention and
control. The precise definition used in any one study is determined
by the type of research that is being carried out, and may draw most
closely from one in particular of the above. Research can aid the
process of cross-fertilisation between different professional groups
and their definitions.

One particular problem with the research definition of which it is necessary to
be aware, is that research subjects in current studies are likely to have been
drawn from groups of those families who have already been labelled child
abusers in legal or medical terms. Hence, the subjects of a research study are
not a representative sample of parents who maltreat their children: they are a
sample of those who have been reported or referred themselves as such, and
who are willing to take part in a research project. As Smith (1984) points out, it
is essential that research reports give details of the exact nature of the sample,
and the way in which it was selected.

Surely, however, the most comprehensive conceptualisation of all should
be the therapeutic one. Perhaps we should ask why we need a definition at all
for this purpose? Certainly, we need definitions which enable us to protect
children against the worst excesses of their parents, and to safeguard life and
limb, but we are in danger of missing a great deal by attaching too much weight
to these. The difficulty in finding workable definitions of emotional abuse,
and the growing realisation that the consequences of this kind of abuse may be
amongst the most profound, requires a degree of reconceptualisation of the
way that we should work with families. We need to be able to detect specific
patterns within individual families which may be working to the detriment of
its members.

THE EMOTIONAL ENVIRONMENT OF THE FAMILY

As we saw earlier, Parton argued that the process of reification led to a
definition of child abuse which was initially comparatively restricted. The use
of a restricted definition is in turn likely to determine the way in which families
are perceived by professional agencies and intervention in families is carried
out. Parton writes:

It is quite apparent that the definitional boundaries of the problem are now very fluid and inconsistent, for the crux of the matter is that non-accidental injury is a socially defined phenomenon and therefore its boundaries cannot be stated as if they were fixed and permanent. Even so it has become a category which is symbolically very powerful.
(Parton, 1979, p. 445)

If this is a problem in the definition of physical abuse, how then can we hope to develop a workable definition of emotional abuse? Studies have concluded repeatedly that the environment in which the child is growing up is likely to have a greater effect than the injury itself, and attempts have been made to take a wider perspective on the kinds of family problems involved. The history of the area of child abuse, however, makes it probable that attempts will be made to conceptualise emotional abuse in the same way that physical abuse has been, with parallel attempts to develop definitions that encapsulate its nature and allow intervention. The study of sexual abuse and help for families where this form of abuse has occurred – an area where at present rapid developments are taking place – is also undergoing the same process. Here, however, there is less likely to be a physically indentifiable, medically recognised set of symptoms, and Finkelhor (1984) discusses the reasons why, as a result, definition and consolidation are likely to be less rapid than has been the case for physical abuse. Although Briere (1984) describes what he terms the Post-Sexual-Abuse Syndrome, or PSAS, this is in fact a long list of many different possible sequelae of abuse. The use of the term 'syndrome' in this context is important, however. Emotional abuse is a yet more difficult, diffuse concept, and thus considerably more difficult to develop adequate definitions for; arguably, the task is too difficult, and practitioners need instead to find other ways of thinking about emotional abuse.

To draw a comparison with the field of psychiatry, Rowe (1978) writes on the search for definitions that capture the nature of depression. She illustrates the difficulties that the psychiatric profession has encountered in trying to devise classifications that cover the range of personal experiences subsumed under this title: up to a dozen different categories at a time can be found in different systems of classification. But, Rowe warns, once the professional accepts a framework of definition, once the process of reification has occurred, a barrier has been set up between the professional's expectations and perceptions and the actual experience of the patient. She writes:

Depression is a name for an experience. If we want to understand what this experience is, how it arises, what it means, and since it is an unpleasant experience, how to avoid it, then we must examine this experience of depression. For every person it is an individual experience, yet when we look we can see something common in all these experiences.
(p. 7)

In the same way, in attempting to come to terms with the emotional abuse of children we need to examine the experience of living together for the families of the children for whom we are concerned. In parallel with Rowe's observations on depression, we are likely to see something common to these families, or to groups of families, which can inform our therapeutic practice. This is perhaps a more fruitful pursuit than the search for ever-better definitions of emotional abuse. This implies a divergence, rather than a convergence, in our conceptualisations of the area. As Rowe points out, in defining an area too closely we may blind ourselves to the experience of those with whom we are trying to work.

In some respects, it may be helpful to approach emotional abuse from another perspective: that of the family. Minuchin, Rosman & Baker (1980) describe the way in which one individual's symptoms may arise as part of a family system which shows certain recognisable patterns of functioning. Focussing on anorexia nervosa, they describe four attributes commonly seen in what they term the anorectic family. These include enmeshment, an extreme form of proximity or emotional intensity in family interaction; overprotectiveness; rigidity, or commitment to the *status quo*; and lack of conflict resolution. In terms of symptomatology, one family member pays a high price for the high level of commitment that family members have to each other, and to maintaining the existing family system. Minuchin *et al.* comment on the blurring of boundaries between subsystems within the family. They comment, too, of the anorectic daughter that 'She is a parent watcher' (p. 59), and further:

The anorectic child tends not to develop the skills necessary for dealing with her own age level. Her overinvolvement with her family handicaps her involvement with the extrafamilial world, causing a developmental lag. Concomitantly, she becomes overly skilled in observing and transacting with adults.   (p. 60)

The parallels with observations of abused children, specifically regarding pseudo-mature behaviour and role reversal, are quite striking here, and it is worth while remembering that Minuchin *et al.* are writing about teenage girls who have not necessarily experienced any form of physical chastisement, let alone abuse; indeed, they may come from families where considerable efforts have been made to avoid any form of conflict.

To take another example, Brown, Birley & Wing (1972), Vaughn & Leff (1976) and others have drawn attention to the relationship between parental style and relapse in young schizophrenic adults. They looked at the quality of comments made by the relatives of schizophrenics during a structured interview, and derived an index of 'expressed emotion' from this. Schizophrenics returning to live with families who exhibited high levels of expressed emotion and who were critical or hostile were at far greater risk of relapse. Emotional overinvolvement was also found to be closely related to relapse. This again suggests strongly that the way in which families express emotion may have far-reaching consequences for individual members. We need, therefore, to attempt to study not only what parents do to their young children, but the way in which the entire family experiences and expresses feelings within its boundaries.

Work on patterns of interaction within the family has begun to suggest ways in which the psychological environment of the abusing family may be studied. Burgess & Conger (1978) found that abusive families not only interacted less, but that when they did interact they were more likely to focus on negative aspects of their relationships. This could perhaps parallel the high frequency of critical comments made by families of schizophrenics studied by Brown *et al.* who had high levels of expressed emotion. A series of studies by Patterson and his colleagues (Patterson & Cobb, 1971; Patterson, 1982) have drawn attention to the ways in which patterns of negative exchanges may develop in families, whilst in a study of marital interaction Gottman (1979) observed consistently occurring sequences of negative exchanges ('negative affect reciprocity') which characterised couples who were reporting marital distress.

Perhaps, therefore, it may be more fruitful to observe the patterns of interactions within families, and to identify sequences of interaction that may become problematic, than to attempt to define what is meant by emotional abuse. This in turn implies that the family, rather than the individual child or parent, should be the focus of intervention.

We have seen so far that the way in which the conceptualisation and definition of child abuse has developed has determined the locus and type of intervention. Both abusing parents and abused children are recognised as needing help, and most recently the family context has been identified as the best area for intervention. Whilst family therapy requires facilities, trained staff and a level of commitment from family members which are not necessarily available where they are needed, the adoption of a perspective which views the family and associated professionals as a system is probably helpful. Beezley *et al.* (1976) noted that abused children could most successfully be helped by psychotherapy when their parents were also willing to change, and to allow their child to change. They also observed that change was more likely in the child if the therapist could bring about changes in the child's daily environment, in a structured day-care setting.

The value of day care for abused children has been emphasised by Mirandy (1976), who points out that it allows the parents respite, provides extra stimulation for the child, allows the remediation of developmental lags, and helps the child to improve social functioning and overcome problematic personality traits. The day-care setting also provides an excellent opportunity for assessment of the child's development and progress in this entire range of domains.

In the next chapter the long-term effects of abuse are considered. Most of the rest of the book describes research and observation at a Family Centre for abused and neglected children and their families, which consisted of a day nursery which the children attended daily and their mothers attended regularly for several days a week. We were there as researchers, not therapists, and used observational and interview approaches to study the development of the children and the nature of their relationships with their mothers. Sadly, we were unable to work with the fathers, who tended not to visit the Centre.

We document here the observational approaches that we used, and attempt to highlight aspects of observation that we found useful in increasing our understanding of these children and their mothers. In particular, we looked at the children's behaviour at play in the nursery, and at the interaction of some of the children and their mothers at mealtimes in the Family Centre. We suggest ways in which these techniques might be used in therapy, in longer-term assessment of the children's development, and in assessment of changes in the mother-child relationship.

We studied a small number of children and their mothers intensively, rather than taking a broad, superficial view of a large number of children, and as such most of the book takes a case-study approach. We feel that in this way we began to identify forms of emotional abuse in some mother–child relationships, and to see its effects on individual children. We were also able to collect some follow-up information on the children's transition to school.

In the chapters that follow we attempt to show the difficulty of defining emotional abuse and adequate levels of care for children, and discuss the ways in which the emotional and physical environment of the child can shape behaviour and development. We show, too, how observational approaches can clarify the present state of the child, and suggest possible areas for intervention. In Chapters 12 and 13 we go on to suggest alternative ways of conceptualising some of the problems of this area, and end with practical suggestions for future research and intervention with abusing families.

2   The long-term effects of child abuse

Arriving at the railway station of Newcastle upon Tyne, one's first impression is of urban decay. 'I always find this place depressing', one fellow traveller commented to me (R.C.). Despite the large and glossy shopping mall, the Metro, and the new bridge over the Tyne, Newcastle carries such a weight of industrial decline and poverty that the problems of the city cannot be concealed.

The flat that I occupied for a year was on the first floor of a small terraced house in a 'respectable' neighbourhood. Downstairs lived a young woman who made her living through prostitution, a trade which folded when she became part of a group of glue-sniffers. My flat developed a heady atmosphere of chemical fumes and loud new wave music, and I took to staying out most evenings. Downstairs also lived the woman's child, a 2-year-old who could be heard crying for hours on end, and who was occasionally found by neighbours, having wandered from home unnoticed. I sometimes found her playing in the snow, wearing no shoes.

The occasional social worker came by. The glue sniffers would disappear silently out of the back window. Social Services told me that the case was under their control and that my comments were not required. Environmental Health came on one occasion and removed the foetid disposable nappies that festered in the house and yard. Eventually, the child disappeared. One of the sniffers told me that she was in care, and had been having treatment for a broken arm – an old fracture. On the day that I moved out, a TV crew were arriving and setting up their equipment to make a documentary on glue sniffing.

How unusual was my neighbour in her treatment of her child? How do levels of child maltreatment in Newcastle compare with those for the rest of England and Wales? This chapter will present the results of a British follow-up study of children placed on the Child Abuse Register administered by the NSPCC around the time of its establishment in the Newcastle upon Tyne region in 1975, and in 1976. A number of the children registered at that time were followed up in the autumn of 1981, at least 5 years after their placement on the Register. Some of the children had been subject to abuse prior to the

15

establishment of the Register, and their injuries date back to 1973 and 1974. Hence, some of the children studied here had been first injured more than 8 years previously. Statistics for the area will be presented, before the study is discussed, in order to give some sense of background to the figures.

CHILD ABUSE IN NEWCASTLE UPON TYNE 1975 AND 1976

Criteria for registration

Children were placed on the Register of Suspected Non-Accidental Injuries to Children if they met the following criteria:

All physically injured children under the age of 16 years where the nature of the injury is not consistent with the account of how it occurred or where other factors indicate that there is a reasonable suspicion that the injury was inflicted or not prevented by any person having custody, charge, or care of the child. In exceptional circumstances, children who have never received a suspected non-accidental injury but are considered to be at serious risk of injury by the notifier may be accepted for registration.

(Annual Statistical Summary, Newcastle Special Unit, 1976)

A comparison with national figures, 1975

The report of the findings of the NSPCC Special Unit Registers for 1975 is of particular value here, as it includes a detailed breakdown of statistics by area. The figures indicate that Newcastle Metropolitan District (MD) had the highest reported rate of injury to under-fives of any Unit in the country: 2.7 per 1000 of the population under 5, compared with a national estimate of 1.5 per 1000. The Newcastle rate for injury to under-fifteens was 0.82 per 1000 of the population under 15, while the national rate was 0.7 per 1000. Compared with figures for other Units, a high percentage of fathers (42.4%) were unemployed.

A comparison with national figures, 1976

Creighton (1980) in the third report on the findings of the NSPCC Special Units reported that the Newcastle area was distinguished by a variety of factors. A higher percentage of low birth weight babies was found, and also a higher proportion of cases of failure to thrive than were registered with other Units. In Newcastle the largest proportion of abused children lived with two natural parents (63.3%), the national figures showing a trend towards abuse being most common in families where there was one natural parent plus a parent-substitute. Newcastle again had the highest proportion of unemployed heads of household (43.3%).

Overall, the national Register figures for 1975 and 1976 indicated that the majority of children suffered only soft tissue injuries. Children less than a year old accounted for the highest percentage of registered cases. Low birth weight babies were over-represented. Parents were characterised by relatively early parenthood, marital discord, non-intact family structure, high mobility and criminality. Creighton (1980) comments:

The children registered in 1976 would appear to come disproportionately from criminal and violent families.

Statistics for Newcastle Metropolitan District, 1976

During 1976, 50 children were placed on the Register for Newcastle MD. This suggested an injury rate of 0.48 per 1000 children in the Metropolitan District when compared with census figures (OPCS, 1977). The registration rate, which included 'at risk' cases, was 0.77 per 1000 children under the age of 15.

At that time Newcastle was operating a Register which covered the Metropolitan Districts of Gateshead, Newcastle, North Tyneside and Northumberland. The children followed up in this study were all from Newcastle MD, the largest contributor to the statistics. Figures will be given for this group only.

Table 2.1. *Injuries to children, Newcastle MD, 1976*

Serious (fractures, head injuries, burns, injestion of toxic substances)	3	(10%)
Moderate (soft tissue injuries)	26	(86.7%)
Failure to thrive	1	(3.3%)
Total	30	
Prodromal (at risk)	20	

In 1976, 30 children in Newcastle MD were registered who showed non-accidental injury (NAI) or failure to thrive. A further 20 were registered as prodromal cases, that is, children considered to be at serious risk of NAI. Table 2.1 shows the breakdown of the nature of injuries for this group. Included in the Register were children who had been injured previously, taken into care before the Register had been established, and who were now about to be sent home. In view of the small number of children included in the figures, any comparison between 1975 and 1976 should be treated with caution.

In 1976, 60% of the injured children were less than 4 years old at the time of the incident. Of the 50 registered children 28 were boys and 22 girls, evenly distributed over the different categories of severity of injury. Forty per cent of the registered children had been injured on a previous occasion.

LONG-TERM EFFECTS: PREVIOUS RESEARCH

What are the effects, in the long term, of these kinds of maltreatment? A few studies have attempted to address this question; however, research to date on the long-term effects of child abuse and neglect has generally suffered from a series of problems. These centre around the definitions of child abuse used, difficulties of experimental design and methodology, and problems inherent in the sample.

Problems of definition

1. 'Child abuse' refers, in different studies, to a wide range of parent–child behaviours. For example, Elmer (1977*a*, *b*) includes children in her comparison groups that on broad criteria would probably be classified as abused.

2. Further, the severity of injury to the child considered varies greatly between studies. A majority appear to refer to children with serious injuries, including fractures and head injuries, although most injuries to children are more moderate. Toro (1982), in a review of the literature, suggests that there is a need to include a wider range of injuries and also neglect of children in order to draw conclusions more directly relevant to the full range of maltreated children.

Problems of experimental design and methodology

1. Jones (1980) comments on the varied sampling techniques used by different studies. Subject recruitment may be via casualty wards, social welfare agencies or juvenile courts. Each source of subjects is likely to carry with it its own characteristics and problems.

2. A lack of matched controls has been noted in many studies (Jones, 1980; Toro, 1982). The choice of appropriate controls is problematic. Elmer (1977*b*) used children who had been admitted to casualty with accidental injuries, and also a second group of carefully matched controls who had been admitted to hospitals with acute infections, as comparisons for children who had suffered NAI. Her results indicated serious family problems within the two comparison groups and also a lack of clear significant differences between these groups and the NAI group. It could be suggested that these control children had been subject to undetected physical abuse, or, at least, to emotional abuse or neglect. Lynch (1976) used siblings of abused children as controls. This group shares to a close approximation the environment of the abused child, but it is possible here, however, that the control sibling may also have suffered NAI which has not been detected. It is essential in planning a control group to be sure what one is controlling.

Problems inherent in the sample

1. *High mobility*. Jones (1980) draws attention to the problems of attempting to trace abused children. Once a family leaves a neighbourhood, records on that child are not maintained unless the child is still considered to be at considerable risk of injury.

2. *Family instability*. Abused children appear to experience high rates of change of family composition, and changes of name associated with this may make children particularly difficult to trace.

3. *Other environmental variables*. It is probable that neglect, rejection and lack of provision of a stimulating environment will accompany physical abuse of the child (Jones, 1980). In attempting to assess the effects of physical injury on children these accompanying variables need to be taken into account.

4. *Social and economic disadvantage*. Further, as both Jones and Elmer point out, social and economic disadvantage are very likely to be associated with abuse and to be major contributors to poor development and performance in assessment tasks. Elmer, discussing her American sample, comments that poverty and membership of a lower class play a major role in determining a child's development, and that the effects of physical abuse may be relatively less significant. Toro (1982) argues for the inclusion of a larger number of middle and upper socio-economic status (SES) children in follow-up studies.

5. *Treatment*. Abused children do not simply show the marks of maltreatment. The sequelae of abuse may vary greatly from child to child. Many are taken into care for periods of varying duration, and may experience multiple changes in caretaking. Separation from the abusing parent also entails separation from a familiar home, with all the implications that carries with it.

Long-term follow-ups: major findings

Readers are referred to Aber & Cicchetti (1983), Cicchetti & Risley (1981), Egeland, Sroufe & Erickson (1983), Jones (1980), Kinard (1982), Martin (1976) and Toro (1982) for a fuller treatment of the literature to date on the long-term effects of abuse on development. Lamphear (1985) also reviews studies in this area. With the major exception of Elmer, studies have tended to indicate a deleterious effect of an abusive environment on the development of children. The evidence available covers neurological status and growth, learning and intelligence, language use and school adjustment. A brief summary of the findings in each area is given below. The effects of abuse on personality are discussed in Chapter 1.

Neurological development, motor activity and growth
Studies of children who have suffered head trauma show evidence of neurological dysfunction (Martin *et al.* 1974, Martin, 1976). There are

indications, however, that these effects can be moderated by placement in a good environment; some of the children in Martin's study were considered retarded, but, with stimulation, developed adequate functioning. Martin (1976) draws attention to Caffey's important work on the effects of shaking on infants, who may develop retardation due to subdural haematoma without showing any physical symptoms. It is possible, therefore, that abused children showing neurological dysfunction may do so as a result of undetected injuries rather than those for which referral was made. Martin *et al.* (1974) noted that children exhibiting failure to thrive were at particular risk of neurological dysfunction, a finding relating problems of this kind to severe and pervasive neglect. Undernourished abused children appear to show poorer developmental outcome than well-nourished abused children (Elmer & Gregg, 1967; Martin *et al.*, 1974). Other authors (see e.g. Lynch, 1976) suggest that growth charts may be a very valuable source of information on the child's continuing development, and that these should form part of long-term assessment wherever possible.

Learning and intelligence

Again, abused children have been found to show deficits in learning and intelligence by some, but not all, studies. For example, Elmer & Gregg (1967), Martin (1976) and Morse, Sahler & Friedman (1970) found that some deficits in intelligence as measured by standard IQ tests. Opposition on the part of the abused child and an unwillingness to attempt the tasks may lead to diminished scores, however, indicating problems of interaction rather than cognition (Lamphear, 1985). In trying to find the causes for lower IQ scores, problems in pregnancy and at birth cannot be excluded. Interpretation of such results therefore requires caution. Neither can physical abuse be seen as the sole cause of such problems, as environmental influences are likely to be major factors. The restriction of opportunities for learning in the abusing family, inadequate stimulation and support, insecurity, danger associated with performance and non-performance and the pre-emption of energies by a need for survival may contribute to poor development (see Martin & Rodeheffer, 1976). However, Lynch (1978) found that 10 years after abuse, 67% of the abused children had IQs of average or above average levels.

Language use

The expressive language skills of abused children have often been found to be poor (Elmer, 1977b). Again, however, environmental influences accompanying abuse are likely to be of major significance. In particular, the caretaker who is not interested in the child is unlikely to spend a great deal of time talking to him or her, and hence there is inadequate input and practice for language skills to be able to develop. Lynch (1978) found language to be seriously affected, verbal IQ also suffering as a result.

School adjustment

Successful adjustment to school in fact involves a set of adjustments on the part of the child: an ability to cope with academic work, to respond well to teachers and the various restraints of the school system, to exercise self-discipline and control, and to form good relationships with peers. This range of requirements makes school adjustment a valuable domain of study.

Some British follow-up studies have used the Bristol Social Adjustment Guide (BSAG: Stott, 1974) in the assessment of abused children. The replication of studies using this tool allows some comparability of data. Roberts *et al.* (1978) followed up 20 abused children and their 25 non-abused siblings at school. The BSAG measures maladjustment along two dimensions: under-reaction, characterised by withdrawn, depressed behaviour, and over-reaction, shown in hostile, deviant and aggressive behaviour. On the dimension of under-reaction the abused children's behaviour was rated as being close to the norm. Roberts *et al.* found, however, that the children had higher levels of over-reaction than might be expected of a normal sample. Around 37% of the abused children and their siblings were showing appreciable to severe maladjustment, hostility accounting for a good deal of this. As regards academic attainment, though, 60% of the children were average or good. Gregory (1981; Gregory & Beveridge, 1984), in a follow-up of a small sample of abused children, also found that adjustment, and not attainment, was the aspect of school functioning that distinguished abused children from their peers. Both Roberts *et al.* and Gregory make one point clear, however; a good percentage of children in both samples were showing satisfactory adjustment; half of Roberts *et al.*'s sample were exhibiting no problems at all.

School adjustment is a particulary useful variable for study in the long-term follow-up of abused children. Firstly, on a practical level, it is a comparatively cheap and rapid way to gain information when compared with paediatric assessments or psychological test batteries. Secondly, it allows an assessment to be made of several aspects of the child's functioning. Thirdly, the assessment need not involve making contact with parents – a potentially difficult and painful procedure, especially with increasing time from last contact with social workers. Fourthly, on a point of methodology, follow-up studies have generally used assessments made by professionals who knew the child's case history. If teachers are not aware of the nature of the study there is some possibility of making a 'blind' assessment of the child, uncontaminated by potential expectations or bias on the part of the assessor.

A FOLLOW-UP STUDY OF SCHOOL ADJUSTMENT

The present study used blind ratings by teachers of the school adjustment of abused children and their peers. Form teachers used the BSAG to evaluate each child's adjustment to the school system, his or her relationships with classmates, and academic attainment.

Using this measure, the progress of some of the children who had been placed on the Register in 1975 and 1976 was followed up (Calam, 1983). The Register is a useful tool for this purpose, as it gives detailed information on family size and composition, periods in care and other changes in caretaking, in addition to information on the nature and severity of injuries leading to referral. It might well be expected that these variables would affect the child's development.

A control group of two non-abused children per abused child was used. These were the boy and girl closest in age to the abused child and in the same class at school. Confidentiality of information was a major concern in setting up the study, and it was therefore essential that the attention of teachers should not be drawn specifically to any one child in the class. Through the use of this kind of control group it was hoped that teachers would not be particularly aware of any one child as the focus of interest. In obtaining information on the children a rather elaborate procedure was employed which ensured that the abused child was not identified as such. The procedure also meant that teachers were blind to the nature of the study as they rated three of their pupils.

The children studied

The names of children currently aged between 5 and 11 years who were attending schools in the Newcastle area and who had been placed on the Register in 1975 and 1976 were obtained from the Community Health Department. Fifty-three children were selected on two criteria: that they were currently living at home and that they were not attending special schools. Clearly, the exclusion of these children in specialised care must lead to a distortion of the results, as these may have been children who had suffered most serious maltreatment. The aim of this study, however, was to gain information on children currently thought to be in satisfactory living conditions and receiving an adequate standard of parental care, having been rehabilitated with their families. To have included children from special schools would also have made the selection of a control group of children difficult. If this subject selection procedure influenced the data in any way, it should have been towards greater conservatism.

Twenty-one girls and 32 boys were included in the initial sample. Injury type ranged from the very severe to minor or unexplained injuries. The distribution of injury differed between the two sexes: the boys had been subject mainly to moderate, soft tissue injuries, while a larger proportion of the girls had been registered with serious injuries including fractures, internal damage and one attempted suffocation.

Obtaining information on the children

As mentioned previously, an elaborate procedure was employed in order to avoid problems of leakage of confidential information. The help of a large number of people was invaluable; the study could not have gone ahead without them. The procedure was as follows:

1.   The names of abused children currently residing in the Newcastle area were provided by the Community Health Department, which also provided a list of the schools that the children were currently believed to be attending.

2.   A letter was sent out to Head Teachers from the Director of Education, telling them that a survey was to be made, and that their cooperation was requested. The nature of the study was not explained.

3.   Education Welfare Officers visited all the schools where a listed child was known to be, and checked the name by which the child was known, also the child's class. At the same time the Officers took the names of the control group from the class register.

4.   Once the correct names of the abused children and the names of the control group were returned, named copies of the BSAG were mailed to the schools, and class teachers were requested to complete and return them as soon as possible. At no point were they told of the nature of the study.

  Most of the forms were returned; information was obtained on 23 abused boys and 15 abused girls. Of the remainder, several had left the area within the previous few weeks. Twenty-two children had changed the name by which they were known; one child had had five changes of name since registration. The returned BSAG forms were then scored, following the instructions set out by Stott (1974).

THE FINDINGS OF THE SURVEY

School attainment

Of the two main measures obtained through the BSAG – school attainment and school adjustment – it appeared that school attainment showed no clear differences between groups. If anything, the abused girls appeared to be performing rather better in reading and arithmetic than were the controls, several receiving high ratings. Tables 2.2 and 2.3 show the data for this comparison, in relation to the BSAG categories of 'good', 'average', 'poor' and 'cannot'. This result, whilst appearing paradoxical at first, may, in fact, be a genuine outcome of the abusive environment. The child must be at far lower

Table 2.2. *Reading ability: percentage per level in abused and control children*

	Abused		Control	
Reading ability	Female	Male	Female	Male
Good	28.6	4.5	22.8	14.3
Average	35.7	40.9	48.6	40.0
Poor	35.7	40.9	25.7	40.0
Cannot	0	13.6	2.9	5.7

Table 2.3. *Mathematical ability: percentage per level in abused and control children*

	Abused		Control	
Mathematical ability	Female	Male	Female	Male
Good	28.6	4.5	22.8	11.4
Average	35.7	54.5	51.5	45.7
Poor	35.7	40.9	25.7	40.0
Cannot	0	0	0	2.9

risk of abuse sitting quietly reading a book than running around, sploshing paint onto paper and clothes, or otherwise creating noise and disturbance. Further, it is possible that high achievement may enhance parental estimation. Hence, by doing well at school and by having sufficient resources to present a good face, these children may have created for themselves a safer environment.

Martin (1976) argues that high achievement by abused children at school need not indicate a healthy adjustment. In his study, 8 of the 58 children showed high IQs in the range 115–131. Martin suggests that the reasons for this include active and intrusive participation in the child's learning by the parents, and probable high valuation of 'being smart' by some parents. Hence, the child who is able to meet the high expectations of parents may avoid harm in this way. High ability may, however, be a trap, Martin argues: 'Children cannot live primarily in a world of books, numbers or thoughts. The child lives primarily in a world of people' (p. 102). Further, Martin noted that high IQ was not associated with a creative or flexible approach to problem solving. These children were hampered on such tests, producing regressive scores. Hence, high intelligence could be used only within limited boundaries.

School adjustment

School adjustment showed clear and disturbing differences between the abused and control children on the dimension of over-reaction, the abused

Table 2.4. *Over-reaction: percentage per level of adjustment in abused and control children*

	Abused		Control	
Over-reaction	Female	Male	Female	Male
Stability and near-stability	57.1	31.8	80.0	68.6
Mild over-reaction	21.4	13.6	5.7	11.4
Appreciable over-reaction	0	4.5	11.4	0
Maladjusted over-reaction	21.4	45.5	2.8	14.3
Severe maladjusted over-reaction	0	4.5	0	5.7

Table 2.5. *Under-reaction: percentage per level of adjustment in abused and control children*

	Abused		Control	
Under-reaction	Female	Male	Female	Male
Stability and near-stability	64.3	63.6	68.6	65.7
Mild under-reaction	0	18.2	5.7	17.1
Appreciable under-reaction	14.3	18.2	14.3	14.3
Maladjusted under-reaction	14.3	0	5.7	0
Severe maladjusted under-reaction	7.1	0	5.7	2.8

children showing significantly higher levels of over-reaction than the control group. This result was statistically significant when tested by analysis of variance ($F = 8.88$, d.f. $= 1.97$, $P < 0.01$). There was also a significant effect of the boys showing a higher level of over-reaction than the girls ($F = 7.42$, d.f. $= 1.97$, $P < 0.01$). Table 2.4 illustrates these data.

These results show very clearly that the continuing progress of a number of the abused group, now no longer under the active care of the local authorities, was not all that might have been hoped. Seven of the abused boys were rated as comparatively stable, 4 were showing mild or appreciable over-reaction, 10 exhibited maladjusted over-reaction, and 1 had severe maladjusted over-reaction. That is, around 45% of the boys were presenting serious behaviour problems in the classroom. The picture for the girls was rather better, only 21% being rated as maladjusted or seriously maladjusted.

Why might this sex difference exist? Izard & Schwartz (1986) suggest on the basis of studies of depressed children, that boys and girls express their depression in different ways. While both show depressed responses on standard measures of the state, boys express their negative feelings in outwardly directed ways, through hostility and aggression. Girls, in contrast, express their unhappiness through low-profile, withdrawn behaviour. Could this be the case for this group of abused children? Did the relationship hold here?

On the dimension of under-reaction, it appeared that there was some difference between the sexes, but little difference between the abused and control children when tested using analysis of variance of the same kind as that used for over-reaction. The figures show that most of the children nestled comfortably into the category of stability/near-stability. What the figures did show, however, was a rather worrying 'tail' of children, specifically girls, and particularly in the abused group, who were showing appreciable to severe maladjustment (Table 2.5). In terms of numbers, the count of cases was small; for the girls concerned, however, this result is worthy of note. Here was a small group of girls, no longer under the care of the authorities, who were showing the kind of withdrawn behaviour that might well be likely to contribute to lack of friendships with peers and, hence, lack of access to positive experiences in one of the most important realms of child development. We do not know, as yet, whether familial violence is transmitted from generation to generation; we do know, however, that one of the key characteristics of many abusing mothers is social isolation and loneliness (Steele & Pollock, 1968). The potential link between these sets of findings could form one of the bases of an attempt to come to terms with a cycle of violence and poor parenting across generations.

The effects of previous experience on school adjustment

Information had been gathered from the Register on the previous experiences of the abused children in the survey. This included information on family composition, the number of changes of caretaker the child had experienced, the duration of periods in substitute care, and the nature, severity and frequency of injuries sustained. All of these might be thought potentially to affect the child's adjustment to school. Was this the case?

In order to find out whether these variables appeared to be having any impact on BSAG scores, each child's score for under- and over-reaction were independently labelled 'satisfactory' or 'poor'. Satisfactory adjustment consisted of scores in the range of stability or near-stability; poor scores were those in the categories of appreciable, maladjusted, and severe maladjusted under- or over-reaction. Statistical tests (Chi square or the Fisher Exact Probability Test) were used to compare school adjustment with previous experience.

Parental status. Children who had been living with a single parent at the time of abuse were considerably more likely to have high over-reaction scores than were those who had been living in a two-parent family ($P = 0.051$), or with a natural parent and parent-substitute ($P = 0.029$). No significant difference was found between the adjustment of children living in two-parent or parent plus parent-substitute families. This may be a result of increased family instability for the children in the one-parent families.

Changes of caretaker. These did not appear to have any significant effect on school adjustment.

Duration of substitute care. Whatever the effects of long-term care, the children in this study who had spent long periods in care did not appear to be showing significantly higher levels of maladjustment than those who had not had this experience. However, children who had experienced short-term care of three months or less showed significantly higher over-reaction scores ($F = 2.99$, d.f. $= 1$, $P < 0.05$). Thus, children who had been taken into care over a comparatively short period as a crisis measure were showing higher levels of maladjustment than those who had stayed at home or those who had returned home after a long period in substitute care. While the number of subjects is small, these results are, perhaps, of importance in their implications.

Injury type and re-injury. This variable did not appear to have any impact on school adjustment scores. This result is important, as it indicates that attention to severity of injury, at the expense of other aspects of the situation at the time the child is referred, may well lead to a range of other factors of potentially far greater significance being ignored.

Other findings

In addition to scoring school adjustment and attainment, teachers rated their pupils on a range of other attributes which are included on the BSAG. Some of the teachers ignored these ratings, which is a pity, as the results that emerge when these apparently less significant variables are considered are most important. What were these attributes?

The BSAG asks teachers to rate children on general appearance, i.e. their perceived attractiveness or apparent lack of it, and also asks for information on general health and a range of defects. For these variables, differences between the abused and control groups again appeared.

Appearance. Teachers were asked to rate children as 'attractive', 'not so attractive' or 'looks undernourished'. They tended not to bother with the 'not so attractive' category, and, for statistical purposes, this was dispensed with. The remaining ratings showed clear differences, the teachers in general classifying more of the abused children as 'looks undernourished' and more of the controls as 'attractive'. Table 2.6 shows these data. So, at least 5 years after abuse, these children, who were now thought to be receiving an adequate level

Table 2.6. *Appearance: percentages by condition and sex*

	Abused		Control	
Appearance	Female (n = 15)	Male (n = 23)	Female (n = 38)	Male (n = 37)
Attractive	57.1	50.0	77.1	57.1
Not so attractive	0	9.0	2.9	8.6
Looks undernourished	21.4	22.7	5.7	8.6
No rating	21.4	18.2	14.3	25.7

of care, were considered to look undernourished. This must surely indicate a continuing level of deprivation, if not neglect. This finding is, of itself, worrying, Worrying too, however, is the probability that these abused children, not rated as attractive by their teachers, might also be less well liked in consequence.

General health and defects. In terms of general health the abused children appeared to be faring less well also, although the difference between the abused and control groups was not significant. Table 2.7 shows the data for this measure. It is worth noting that 35% of the abused children and 18.6% of controls were reported to be suffering frequent health problems. As regards defects, too, the abused children were showing a higher percentage than the controls. These results again suggest that these children were continuing to receive an inadequate level of care.

Informal comments by teachers

In addition to the information formally requested by the BSAG, a space was provided on the form for other comments that the teacher might like to make. Teachers made comments on 9 of the abused children, and on 9 of the controls. These comments are reproduced verbatim in Table 2.8, as they give some indication of the variation within the groups of children.

It is notable, first of all, that almost all of the comments elicited by this part of the BSAG dwelt on the children's problems. For the abused children, only one of the comments was wholeheartedly positive in tone; the figure for the control children was two. The teachers commented on a far larger proportion of the abused children than the controls. With regard to the content of the comments, it would be difficult to attempt to distinguish those for the abused and the control children. One comment on one of the abused girls, Jan, does stand out however. From the teacher's description, Jan is a neglected child, and has a need, real or imagined, to conceal aspects of her home life from her teacher and classmates. Other children in the control group are also living with

Table 2.7. *Poor health and defects: percentages by condition and sex*

	Abused		Control	
	Female	Male	Female	Male
Poor health	42.9	27.3	11.7	25.7
Physical defect	14.3	27.3	5.7	17.1
Speech or language defect	0	31.8	2.9	25.7

Table 2.8. *All informal comments made by teachers on the BSAG*

Abused group: boys

'A quiet, well-behaved little boy who enjoys the company of his peers and is gaining confidence all the time. I expect his work to develop from average to good because of his attitude and perseverance.'

'Barry tries very hard but has very limited ability.'

'Extenuating home circumstances – lives with aunt instead of mother. In spite of everything, he is coping pretty well.'

'Child is "in care", but living with his brother after a court case this year.'

'Most of Colin's antisocial behaviour occurs out of the classroom although often in school – in school playground etc. There is almost the expectancy of trouble with him.'

Control group: boys

'In my view he has much ability and is seriously under-achieving.'

'Pointless having face to face confrontations with Billy; he becomes impossible. He has to be coaxed and flattered into working and behaving. Can produce neat work. Poor academically however.'

'Graham can be a pleasant boy, but he spoils himself by being spiteful towards weaker children, especially if he feels he might get away with it. Will often incur the wrath of older children through his spitefulness and then complain that he is being "picked on".'

'Specific reading difficulties. Father has apparently had a long period in hospital. John's behaviour in this school has been mainly irritating, not seriously disruptive. Diagnostic reading tests have been arranged and his father is now at home. Perhaps this will effect an improvement in his attitude.'

'On rare occasions Tony shows interest. He is capable of imaginative stories and much improved general attitudes. Tony comes from a one-parent family. His mother is over-critical and treats Tony as an adult in certain situations. She discusses problems and is inclined to dwell on the morbid. Tony seems to "switch off" to this and this could be much to do with the attitudes outlined in the test.'

Table 2.8 (cont.)

Abused group: girls	Control group: girls
'Joanne enjoys school and is of above average ability. Her only problems seem to be those of chattering at every possible opportunity and the odd disagreement with a classmate (usually initiated by Joanne). Tendency to boss her immediate peer group.'	'Sally is very artistic and has produced some beautiful work. Creative.'
	'Amy is a pleasant hardworking girl who always gives her best.
'There is an air of neglect about Jan, but nothing that can be pinpointed. For example, she has curly hair but it never looks combed. She is very secretive about her home – in group discussions, for instance, she won't say what she had for breakfast.'	'Although sometimes restless and too talkative, generally speaking this little girl can be channelled towards acceptable behaviour both in and out of the classroom.'
'Very sensitive. Tiny and underweight. Children are being monitored for this.'	'Mandy has abnormal control for a child of her age. Seems an unhappy child. Is supposed to be very badly behaved at home. We have never seen this side of her.'
'Marie suffers considerably from eye trouble. She has, on a number of occasions, been to hospital for tests, which has been responsible for Marie's prolonged absence from school. A pleasant girl in normal conversation, but extremely timid.'	

considerable problems, and, in two cases, the teachers make specific reference to poor family dynamics in order to explain the child's problems.

This study picked up a number of children who, registered or not, were suffering neglect and emotional abuse, if not physical injury or sexual abuse.

AN OVERVIEW OF THE STUDY FINDINGS

It would appear from this long-term follow-up that the abused children as a group were more prone to a range of behaviour problems, poor general health and appearance than were their non-abused controls. The abused boys in particular were distinguished by the high percentage of serious behaviour problems, which took such forms as attention-seeking behaviour, hostility, deviance and defiance. The girls, who had, in general, been more severely injured, were showing lower levels of maladjustment. Again, this provides evidence that attention to injury *per se* rather than other aspects of the situation may lead to important factors being overlooked. It may be that these girls had experienced a more concerted intervention by social services as a result of their injuries, in which case their judgement scores are an optimistic note. Not optimistic, however, were the scores for almost half the boys, nor those for the girls showing maladjusted over- and under-reaction.

Many of the children in the study were presenting no problems at all. At the same time, however, a substantial proportion of the control group were also showing problems. It may well be the case, as Elmer (1977b) suggests, that the social milieu of deprivation should be considered a powerful influence on the developing child, aside from physical injury. But differences *were* found between the abused and control children, indicating that they were experiencing a particularly poor level of continuing care. This study cannot offer information on the relative influences of deprivation, poverty, familial style of interaction and physical abuse on children. Were there measures of less dramatic and less easily classifiable forms of maltreatment readily available, it is likely that a control group could have been selected that showed levels of maladjustment as severe as those of the abused children. If we have the interests of children at heart, we should be attempting to identify those other forms of maltreatment, and to treat them seriously.

Some overlapping evidence

One particular study is of considerable relevance when considering the data arising from this long-term follow-up. Speight, Bridson & Cooper published a study in 1979 reporting a rather shorter-term follow-up of the health and development of children abused in Newcastle in 1974 and 1975. Their report is of particular significance when compared with the results reported here on children abused around that time in the same city; some of the children whose scores are reported here were probably in Speight *et al.*'s study. Speight *et al.* suggested that relatively minor NAI in this sample was an index of serious family pathology; many of the children were chronically deprived. They argued that neglect and deprivation in their sample had probably been under-diagnosed and under-managed and that the neglect suffered by the children was probably far more significant in terms of long-term development than the isolated incidence of NAI would suggest. They commented that doctors and social workers, preoccupied with physical injury, failed to take other forms of maltreatment into account. Developmental and emotional assessments were, they stated, conspicuous by their absence in reports on the children. Many of the children, they argued, needed to be in care, but that would only occur if there were a proven case of NAI. Speight *et al.* listed five areas in which they considered the management of these child abuse cases to be sub-optimal. These were:

1.   Failure to recognise poor growth, neglect and deprivation.
2.   Failure to treat the above with sufficient seriousness.
3.   Faulty decision making leading to re-injury.
4.   Ill-advised rehabilitation in the family leading to re-injury.
5.   Failure to provide early family placements for long-term care.

As the results of our long-term follow-up carried out in 1981 showed, the continuing development of many of the abused children was not encouraging.

SOME IMPLICATIONS

The present study indicates, we believe, a significant and disturbing level of poor adjustment within this group of abused children, particularly the boys. Such data are probably important, but are rarely collected. How might the task of follow-up be made easier? Firstly, good, accurate record-keeping on each child, centrally maintained, is essential. Whilst there is always alarm at the thought of computerisation of records, a central computer bank of information on abused children could be of great value and significance in attempting to maintain long-term information. Secondly, the BSAG is a useful tool, liked by teachers (Roberts *et al.*, 1978) and easy to use. An annual follow-up of abused children in school would be a comparatively cheap procedure, and could be made part of routine reviews of abused children prior to deregistration.

A central problem is that of funding. Concern over child maltreatment will have to focus on injury and crisis support for as long as those that control the purse-strings see other forms of maltreatment as unimportant. The follow-up reported here should be a cause for concern; at least half of the boys studied were difficult, deviant and hostile. How this might be translated into adolescent and adult behaviour is open to conjecture.

There is a problem in reporting a study of the kind discussed here. The child's deviance appears a *school* problem, but in fact it is a social problem, with, it is clear, long-term consequences; its origins were commented on with alarm by Speight *et al.* some time ago. If we can see a source of deviance, violence and aggression, surely it is more efficient, never mind humane, to attempt to cope with this in its infancy? Roberts *et al.* (1978) make two clear policy-related statements which are relevant here. Firstly, school entry is not an end to the problem of child abuse, although some of the worst manifestations may be ameliorated. Teachers can be made aware of difficulties, and their relationship with the child can form an important part of a continuing therapeutic intervention. Secondly, Roberts *et al.*'s follow-up, and others reported here, indicate clearly that abused children need and deserve treatment in their own right. It cannot be assumed that children will absorb the effects of intervention with parents. A similar point is made by Jones (1980):

It is becoming increasingly apparent that 'therapeutic optimism' is simply not justified in some cases, and that children should not be left in limbo while long drawn out efforts are made to change or modify their parents' attitudes and behaviour.   (p. 152)

What, then, are the variables, aside from physical injury, that merit attention? How may 'good enough' parenting be defined and assessed? The children in this study were, presumably, assumed to be receiving adequate parenting, yet the development of a large proportion of them was far from satisfactory. What kinds of continuing problems might they be experiencing at home? The following chapters document case studies of a group of abused children and their mothers attending a centre for abusing families. The study of these families helps to clarify the answers to these questions.

3   *Working in the Family Centre*

In 1981 and 1982 the authors worked at a Family Centre which dealt exclusively with the families of children who had been physically or emotionally abused, neglected, or who were failing to thrive. The Centre was located on the lower floors of a building housing a team of NSPCC social workers, who thus had easy access to the children. We, as research psychologists, were invited into the Family Centre with the aim of providing additional information on the families to that which had already been obtained through the usual social work and Family Centre channels or was known from other professional sources. Cristina Franchi worked at the Centre in 1981 (Franchi, 1982), and Rachel Calam a year later in 1982. We were hoping to be able to make some contribution to the formidable battery of expertise already available in this setting.

Our aim was to use our particular training to collect information on different aspects of the parent–child relationship from those with which the social work, medical and nursery practitioners were used to dealing. We realised, early on, that in order to provide useful information we needed to work intensively with a small sample of children, and to develop measures aimed at a specific age-range. We eventually chose to work with the 3- to 4-year-olds, selecting these as a group that was using language and hence amenable, at least in principle, to a range of tests and measures which could not have been used with babies. This age-range also enabled peer interaction to be usefully studied.

In all, we were able to collect data on 11 children, from 9 families. Because of the comparatively long time base of our research, we were able to collect information on some families over a 2-year period, picking up younger siblings as they entered the age-range of our study. Before beginning to talk about the individual families, we need to describe the Family Centre, its aims and ideals, the routine of the nursery, the staff there, then the children and their mothers. Lastly, we outline our role as researchers, and the particular constraints that the setting of the Family Centre placed upon us.

THE SETTING FOR THE RESEARCH: THE FAMILY CENTRE

The Family Centre was a specialised social work provision for abusing families and their children. These families were on the caseloads of NSPCC Senior Social Workers, who occupied a suite of offices above the Family Centre and who carried out intensive casework with these families. The Matron and her staff (a deputy and three Nursery Officers) had places for up to 20 pre-school children and their parents. Mothers, and sometimes fathers too, each attended for two days a week on Mondays, Tuesdays, Thursdays and Fridays. The children attended five days a week, Wednesdays being a 'mother-free' day. All the children and most mothers were transported to and from the Family Centre by taxi. (Some children were in care and did not live with their parents. These mothers made their own way to the Family Centre.) There were two taxi runs each morning and afternoon: the first taxi run arrived at the Centre at 10.00 a.m. and left again at 3.00 p.m.; the second arrived at 11.00 a.m. and left at 4.00 p.m. Thus the day's full complement of mothers and children were present between 11 a.m. and 3 p.m.

The accommodation consisted of a mothers' room with the Matron's office and a bathroom off to one side, the babies' room (a double room which was used as the babies' nursery and for meals), a kitchen, a laundry room and a children's bathroom. A ramp led down from the mothers' room, past a small area used for private conversations, to the downstairs playroom, where the 2- to 4-year-olds played. There was also an outside play area, which could be reached from both the downstairs playroom and the babies' room.

Broadly speaking, the day's routine was as follows. On arrival the children were given a drink and a biscuit. They were then taken down to the children's bathroom to be toileted and changed; those mothers present were responsible for their own children at this time, the other children being looked after by the nursery staff. The older children then went to the downstairs playroom or, weather permitting, to the outside play area. The babies were kept in the babies' room or, if their mothers were present, in the mothers' room. Lunch was served from 12 to 12.45 p.m. in the babies' room; mothers were responsible for their own children at such times. The mothers then returned to their room and the children to their playrooms. Mothers were responsible for changing their children before going home. Tea was served at 2.45 p.m. in the babies' room, generally for the children only.

The daily routine and the timing of the taxi runs did impose some constraints on the times research could usefully be carried out. However, despite these constraints the usefulness of the Family Centre as a setting for research should not be minimised. It could be regarded as a naturalistic setting for this sample group. Children could be observed in a free play setting five days a week, their mothers being present for two of these days. A mother-free day on Wednesday meant the children were available for more extended testing, and mother–child interaction at lunchtime could be observed on two days a week for each mother–child dyad.

THE NURSERY STAFF

The philosophy of the nursery staff was to provide a warm atmosphere of re-parenting for all: for the mothers, in the hope of making up for the emotional poverty that many had suffered throughout their lives, and for the children, so that they might be able to develop in a loving atmosphere, in which emotional damage arising from their home environment might be ameliorated.

The maintenance of this atmosphere made the nursery staff's job difficult in some respects in relation to the mothers. This was particularly so when children came in in the morning with a new injury. The non-judgemental warmth of the Centre also meant that the staff found it difficult to act when a mother chastised a child too firmly, either physically or verbally. The hope was that the mothers would learn through observation the ways in which their children could best be disciplined; children were never smacked by staff in the Family Centre. Examples later in the book will show the ways in which the staff controlled the children. The staff disciplined the children discreetly and in an overriding atmosphere of warmth which relied heavily on the resourcefulness of the Nursery Officers and their commitment to the children. The difference between the behaviour of the staff and that of some of the mothers towards the children could not have been more extreme, yet the staff succeeded in maintaining an understanding and forgiving environment.

THE CHILDREN

The children will be discussed in so much detail in the rest of the book that little need be said here. Each morning they ran from the taxi into the arms of the nursery staff, and fell into the daily routine. They played indoors or out, depending on the weather, and superficially appeared to be well cushioned from the darker aspects of their lives. To visitors making a quick tour of the Family Centre, a peep into the playroom showed a happy group of busy children. Closer observation revealed that much of this was attributable to the resourcefulness of the nursery staff, who kept the children occupied at all times, often with the clear intention of avoiding fights. Systematic observation revealed yet more problems that individual children were attempting to cope with. Keith rode round on a bicycle, apparently happily occupied, but observation revealed that this was almost at the level of a compulsion, and associated with anxious monitoring of the environment. Alan was adept at sneaking up to staff without being noticed, so that he could monitor their behaviour. Carl often guarded his little brother to the exclusion of any form of play.

THE MOTHERS

Although one of the stated aims of the Family Centre was to encourage good parenting practices amongst the mothers, the mothers clearly relished the opportunity of having caring, skilled staff around to look after their children for them. So, rather than taking an active role in the care of their children in the Family Centre, the mothers sat back in the central entrance area, where there were comfortable chairs, a carpet, television and many ashtrays, and, in a pall of smoke, discussed their lives with one another.

In this atmosphere, it was our impression as observers that a strong culture was maintained by the mothers which the Nursery Officers had difficulty in making an impact upon. One shared assumption was that the mothers did not do anything with their children unless specifically told to. This amounted to a consistent institutionalised neglect of the children by their mothers. The only time that mothers and children could be seen sitting together was at mealtimes, when the mother's attendance was compulsory. As Chapter 6 will show, the mothers in this setting generally ignored their children or made misguided attempts to control them, and the speed with which some mothers ate their meals and then deserted their offspring was very noticeable.

The mothers frequently mentioned their children in conversation in the mothers' room, but their comments tended to be highly derogatory, and often reinforced by the other mothers. Hence Connie commented of her 3-month-old baby that she was a devil, always going out of her way to be naughty, and the others agreed. Often, their children's naughty behaviour was blamed on the Family Centre: 'he learnt that in here'. The children were not the only targets of scorn. Husbands and boyfriends were daily demolished, and the impression given was that all men were the same: dishonest, drunken, and out for what they could get.

Another area of concern to us was the way in which the group of mothers condoned the use of drugs; several were on tranquillisers, and it was generally agreed amongst the group that this was a good way to get through the day. Conversations focussed on the best tranquilliser to take, rather than on the utilisation of personal resources in dealing with problems.

THE FATHERS

We had hoped to include the children's fathers in the research study, but none of them attended the Family Centre. Whilst some were working, the main reason for non-attendance appeared to be a feeling that child care was the responsibility of the mother, and the Family Centre routine had evolved in such a way that men would probably have had difficulty fitting in. For this reason, we cannot include any information on the fathers other than that which we obtained from the mothers and the Family Centre staff and casefiles, unfortunate as the resulting imbalance may be.

The sample consisted of 11 pre-school children and their 9 mothers; each of the children had been placed on the NSPCC Register as cases or siblings of cases of non-accidental injury (NAI) or suspected NAI (see Chapter 2 for criteria of registration). All were involved in social casework and great care had to be taken not to upset established social work relationships or the equilibrium of the family. It was therefore agreed from the outset that if either mother or child became at all distressed in the course of the research, then that particular research exercise would be discontinued immediately. Similarly, it was agreed that a mother's refusal to cooperate would be accepted without question. It was hoped, however, that the full cooperation in the research of both mothers and children could be obtained without causing distress to any party. An immediate approach was thus ruled out, as the likely response would have been refusal to cooperate.

From the research point of view, this meant that a lot of time had to be spent fitting into the routine of the Family Centre and allowing the mothers and children to become accustomed to the observer.

Unknown, or little-known, adults do not go unnoticed in the Family Centre. The mothers are very sensitive to the presence of strangers and are aware that their attendance at the Centre in some ways identifies them as 'bad' mothers. To avoid fuelling the mothers' feelings of inadequacy, each observer had to establish herself as a non-threatening person before she could begin to work with them. Working with the children was used as a 'way in', but the children as the focus of the observer's attention had to be balanced from a mother's point of view by a genuine interest in her and her problems. These mothers can be characterised as very attention-seeking, looking for much reinforcement and positive feedback in any social interaction – a point which affected the role of the observer.

The children also, after initial apprehensions, enjoyed adult attention and actively sought it out. Before any research could be carried out with them, the observer had to allow them to become used to her presence so that she could, if necessary, withdraw from the situation without upsetting them or persuade the children to leave the playroom with her. It was also necessary, therefore, for the observer to be a familiar figure in the playroom before she could attempt to record peer interaction.

A week was spent interacting with the children in the playroom much as the nursery staff do, and this was followed by a week carrying out trial observations. Initially, the children were very interested to know what the observer was doing as she sat in a corner, pad in hand or bleeper in ear. The observer explained that she was 'working' and that she would play with the children when she had finished. After a few days of the observer collecting trial observations for 10- or 20-minute stretches morning and afternoon, the children accepted that, when in her 'observer' stance, she was not available for play or caretaking. If the target child or any other child approached, the observer gave a minimal response, often just a smile. The staff cooperated in seeing that children did not approach the observer when she was recording, explaining that she was 'working', and in seeing that, as far as was possible, the target child was not removed from the playroom once recording had begun. Occasionally it was necessary to remove a child for toileting, but efforts were made to keep the time of absence to a minimum.

This approach became so accepted by everyone at the Family Centre that when the observer began recording mother–child interaction at lunchtime, no one betrayed the least interest except to ask if she was not going to have any lunch!

CONTROL GROUP

Much consideration was given to the question of a control group. With such a small abused sample it was not possible to control for the specific nature and extent of the abuse suffered by the child. We were also keen to collect data without initially knowing the specific circumstances that had led to the family's attendance at the Centre. What was known about the families' circumstances (for example, the variable presence or absence of the father, the mother's involvement in prostitution, etc.) indicated that finding matched controls might be difficult. It was not possible to control for the nature or degree of abuse in the abused group, and to control for absence of abuse in a matched control group would not have been easy. Abused children and their families do not form homogenous groups and since psychological research on this group is so much in its infancy, it was felt that a control group was not essential. Siblings of abused children were, however, included. Our aim was to develop measures which might best characterise behaviour and interaction in individual mother–child dyads, and within the group of children, making the fullest possible use of the research opportunities offered by the very special setting of the Family Centre.

4 Interview and observational techniques

In embarking upon this research we were well aware that knowledge of the individual histories of the children we were studying was likely to influence the kinds of information that we gathered on them during observation, however good our intentions. For this reason we carried out the majority of our observational work before collecting biographical and interview data on the children. For ease of presentation in this book, however, we discuss our results in a more logical sequence, giving background information on the children and findings from interviews in Chapter 5, and then going on to discuss the results of our observational work in Chapters 6 to 8. The discussion in this chapter of the methods used also follows this sequence.

The sources of information that we used in studying the children and their mothers were as follows:

1. Casefiles and unstructured interviews with the nursery staff.
2. A structured maternal interview drawn from Newson & Newson (1968), and after Light (1979).
3. Observation of the children and their mothers at lunchtime.
4. Observation of the children's activity, peer interaction and hostility.
5. Observation of the children's approach, reaction, approach-avoid-ance and hostility.

An important aspect of psychological assessment is the ability to select the system of behavioural descriptors which best addresses the specific problems that are under investigation. The authors worked independently at the Family Centre, approximately one year apart. Whilst the interview schedule used was the same throughout, the techniques employed for observation were different, reflecting our different interests. This means that while we do not have strictly comparable observational data on all children, we are able to describe a wider range of possible alternative observation techniques and settings. The intensive use of these systems over an extended period gives us confidence in the validity of these techniques for use with this type of sample.

BACKGROUND AND INTERVIEW MATERIAL

Casefiles and information from nursery staff

At the end of our research periods at the Family Centre, each of us read through the casefile for each child in the sample, making a record of major events in the family's life, and collecting as much information as possible on the child's background and experiences. Also at this time, we interviewed the Matron of the Family Centre and collected a great deal of additional information on the child's background, and the individual characteristics of each child and mother. In addition we found that we collected a considerable amount of information, often in the form of anecdotes, by chatting informally to the nursery staff.

Maternal interview

The interview schedule for 4-year-olds developed and used extensively by Newson & Newson (1968) and also after Light (1979), was employed as the basis for the collection of information from the mothers on the children at home. This covers such areas as independence, independence in play, aggression in play, autonomy in play, meals, personal habits, bedtime, toilet training, general discipline, babysitting and changes in upbringing. (For the full interview schedule see the Appendix.)

The section on fathers' participation that formed part of the original interview schedule was omitted for this sample group: some mothers were on their own, some had cohabitees, who were not necesssarily the children's fathers, and some were married. Relationships with men appeared to be a problem for these women and we did not want to get over-involved in this area. References to 'Daddy' or other adults helping with the children were already included in questions in the other sections and it was felt that in the circumstances the information from these would be adequate. Some questions on background from the original schedule were also omitted: some of the information was forthcoming anyway, the rest was obtained later from the Matron's casefiles. The interviews were audiotaped. The order of the questions set out in the interview schedule was largely adhered to, but if a mother spontaneously went on to a different section the interviewer followed her lead, being careful to return to omitted sections later. The questions were 'open-ended', with probe questions inserted as appropriate.

There were problems inherent in administering a maternal interview to this particular sample; the very fact of their attendance at the Family Centre defines them as abusing mothers, that is 'bad mothers', and some questions asked were very obviously designed to probe their mothering skills. The interviewer conducted the interviews 'blind', that is with no knowledge of the circumstances that had led to the families being referred to the NSPCC, so the chance of an unconscious stress being applied to any particular question, or an unconscious reaction being given to any of the replies, was minimised. The interviewer was at pains to put the mothers at their ease. Inevitably some did find the situation a little threatening, but on the whole they all appreciated the opportunity to talk to someone in a one-to-one situation. It was difficult to adhere to a strict interviewer role, as it proved necessary to provide more interactional support and positive feedback in the interview than one would normally expect to in administering a questionnaire. The interviewer tried to keep her verbal response to a minimum but did react positively to what a mother said. She strove to stress her interest in what that particular mother did or thought and tried not to give any impression that there might be a right or a wrong answer, in an attempt to deter the mothers from saying what they thought the interviewer wanted to hear.

OBSERVATIONAL TECHNIQUES

The collection of behavioural data by direct observation

Direct observation has certain advantages over other methods of collecting data such as interviews. It helps to avoid the possibility of discrepancies between real and reported behaviour and does not depend on the verbal capacities or cooperation of the subject. With this sample it was recognised that particular mothers might be uneasy or not very forthcoming about describing how they interacted with their children. Observation of mother–child interaction at lunchtimes was intended to be a valuable complement to maternal interview data, and observations of the children in the playroom provided information about how the children themselves behaved.

The presence of an observer in these situations, however, demands decisions as to what her or his level of participation is to be. In any social setting the presence of an observer must be assumed to have some disruptive effect, although it is usually not possible to measure the size and nature of this directly. Depending on location the options are:

1. *Covert observation:* from behind a one-way screen. These conditions are normally only available in a laboratory setting although, increasingly, nurseries are being designed to include this facility. Young children are not usually aware that they are being watched from behind a mirror and therefore their behaviour is unlikely to be affected. Adults are much more likely to realise that they may be under observation.

2.   *Non-participant observation*: being physically present but remaining silent and refusing to interact with the child. In classroom or day nursery settings it has been shown that children habituate fairly rapidly to the presence of a non-participating observer (Connolly & Smith, 1972; Hughes *et al.*, 1979).

3.   *Participant observer*: being physically present but speaking only when spoken to directly by the child who is the target of the observation. This option is often adopted if the observation is to be carried out in the home. Dunn & Kendrick (1980) maintain that it is inevitable that the presence of an observer will affect interaction of family members. However, from longitudinal studies (Richards & Bernal, 1972; Dunn & Wooding, 1977) it appears that the child's behaviour does not become particularly conforming or obedient, although it may initially involve friendly overtures to the observer, and mothers tend to treat the observer in a very relaxed way and are too busy with housework and child care to change their habitual styles of coping during the many hours the observer is present in the home.

4.   *Action research*: interacting normally with the child who is the target of the observation. The observer has a dual role as both active participant in interactions and recorder of those interactions (Sandow, 1979). Under these conditions the scoring of behavioural data may have to be performed *post hoc*.

The Family Centre was considered to be a fairly naturalistic setting for the sample group, and the observer necessarily had to be present. (The Centre did not at that time have facilities for covert observation of mothers or children.) It was decided that non-participant observation was not appropriate with this sample: a totally non-participant observer carrying out observations in the playroom might have caused the children to become distressed.

Open versus closed systems in observation

Many different approaches can be used in observing children. Where the researcher is unsure what she or he is likely to find in studying an individual or group, but knows that something interesting and important is happening, an excellent starting point is to make as full a record as possible of everything that is going on, and then to examine and extract meaning from this record later. The availability of comparatively cheap videotape recording facilities has led to a great expansion in the detailed study of interaction. Even with videotape, however, it is necessary to find ways of partitioning, abbreviating and summarising the stream of behaviour in order to describe patterns and sequences, and to allow comparability between subjects. Where videotape facilities are not available, and such was the case in the Family Centre, the observer must develop techniques for providing an abbreviated record of behaviour before starting to observe.

A first technique is to observe and take shorthand notes without any preconceived notion of what is going to be found. We describe this as an '*open*' system, as the observer is free to include anything that is going on and appears important. Thus the observer watches a particular child, generally within some time structure, and notes down through a set of abbreviations all that is going on. A next stage following from this is the classification of behavioural units using categories of behaviour, and in this way the shorthand notes describing the stream of behaviour are transcribed into a series of behavioural categories. The combination of shorthand recording with a specific system of behavioural categories is a very useful one, in that it allows the observer all the benefits of the use of a category system while at the same time providing a description of the behaviour in which the child is engaged, thus allowing re-analysis or interpretation at a later date. It is, however, laborious to use, as the transcription of the shorthand into a set of codes takes additional time.

Where the observer has a clear hypothesis about some aspect of the sample which he or she wishes to test, then a more limited, or '*closed*' system of categories allows a specific test to be made of that hypothesis. The observer develops a set of specific categories, designated by particular symbols, and then makes a record only of the occasions on which the child who is being observed is engaged in those particular behaviours. Only a particular set of codes can be used and other behaviour, however interesting, not falling within the set categories is not recorded.

In the research described in this book both open and closed systems were used: observations of lunchtime and some of the peer interactions were conducted using a shorthand system which was later transcribed and coded, while the study of approaches and approach-avoidance was carried out using a closed system of categories. As the following chapters will show, each system has its own strengths, depending on the type of problem to which it is applied.

MOTHER–CHILD INTERACTION AT LUNCHTIME

The observations on mother–child interaction at lunchtime were carried out on the first set of mother–child pairs studied, towards the end of the 1981 period of research at the Family Centre. The way that the mothers would react to having the researcher present and observing during this part of the day was not known, and this form of observation was carried out last in order not to jeopardise the collection of other information on the children. In fact, the presence of an observer at lunchtime was accepted without question. Ten observation periods were recorded, two for each child; in each case one session was on a day that the mother was present, and the other on a day when she was absent. The observational techniques used were the same as those for the peer interaction described in the next section, and will therefore not be discussed here.

The observer carried out the observations in the Family Centre babies' room at lunchtimes. Just before lunch she took a seat in a corner which enabled her to see what was going on at the two lunch tables. Recordings of the target pair began at the moment that the child came in and sat down at a table, and were continued for the whole of that particular lunchtime (lunchtimes varied from 14.5 to 23 minutes in length). A time base was provided by a 30-second electronic bleeper, and data were recorded on the same sheets as used for the peer observations. Each 30-second period on the sheets was bisected horizontally by a dotted line; the child's behaviour was recorded in the upper half and the mother's/adult's behaviour in the lower half.

PEER INTERACTION

Both of the authors studied peer interaction in the same setting: either the Family Centre playroom or outside play area, the weather determining the location. Both also took one focal or target child at a time, and for a set period made continuous observations of the stream of behaviour in which that child was involved. In 1981 a comparatively stable population was available at the Family Centre, so that each child could be observed for an equal amount of time. In 1982 this could not be achieved. Three of the seven children being studied went into and came out of care in the five-month period of study, and one mother only gave permission for her child to take part late on in the research. The mothers of this second group were also, in general, far less regular attenders at the Family Centre.

Observation of activity, peer interaction and hostility

In 1981, each of 5 children was observed for a total of 120 minutes; a target child was observed continuously for 20 minutes under each of the following conditions:

1.   Mother present, in the morning.
2.   Mother present, in the afternon.
3.   Mother absent, in the morning.
4.   Mother absent, in the afternoon.
5.   Wednesday morning (no mothers present at all).
6.   Wednesday afternoon (no mothers present at all)
(The terms 'present' and 'absent' refer to the mother's attendance or not at the Family Centre, not her presence or absence in the playroom.)

Children were allocated to particular sampling days at random. Data for mornings and afternoons were not collected on the same day. Data was not collected on a child if something had happened to upset that child prior to arrival at the Family Centre (for example temporary removal to foster care), or if he or she failed to settle in the Centre and appeared overly upset or withdrawn.

Data were collected in the morning from 11.15/11.30 a.m. to 11.35/11.50 a.m., depending on which taxi the child had arrived in. Data collection was not started until all the children had arrived, and the target child was allowed at least 15 minutes to settle in to the Centre (after caretaking, etc.). In the afternoon, data were collected between 1.15/1.30 p.m. and 1.35/1.50 p.m. (thus allowing half an hour to elapse after lunch) and between 2.00/2.15 p.m. and 2.20/2.35 p.m. if two lots of data were to be collected in one afternoon.

Data were noted down on prepared sheets. Each 30-second period on the sheets was divided in half horizontally by a dotted broken line, the child's behaviour being recorded in the upper half and any responses to or initiations to the child by others in the lower half. A continuous line separated one 30-second period from the next. Five minutes' worth of data were recorded on each sheet (see Figure 4.1).

Piloting of behaviour categories to be recorded was carried out first in the University Nursery and then at the Family Centre nursery during the second week of the researcher's attendance. During the piloting in the Family Centre it was noted that the children tended not to spend long uninterrupted periods at one activity but instead often approached adults for attention, changed activities, wandered around the play area and were involved in hostile exchanges with other children. It was decided, therefore, to record a target child's behaviour in full, much as Sylva, Roy & Painter (1980) did, rather than initially to use discrete and predefined behaviour categories. Boxes on the right of the recording sheets enabled the observer to note down the type of social involvement, play activity and hostility, but on the whole this analysis was carried out when the recordings were transcribed later on the same day. The continuous recording was done using a shorthand notation of common behaviours, with any additional information and scraps of dialogue being noted down in longhand.

Transcription and analysis of data
The categories used for analysis were adapted from Manning, Heron & Marshall (1978) and were used to score types of activity, social involvement and hostility. Whenever possible these categories were recorded directly at the time, otherwise they were reconstructed from the shorthand notes following transcription. The categories, which are defined and described in Table 4.1, include different forms of play, namely active play, manipulative

Fig. 4.1. Example of part of a recording and its transcription.

Subject: Kevin   Date: 18.6.81   am/~~pm~~   Mother ~~present~~/absent

Incidents		Social involvement	Types of activity	Hostility	State*
Riding bike	L.A.	pp	ap	—	
0.5					
Riding bike Loc's	Loc(Sally)voc's LA	pp	ap	—	
1 min					
on bike	Loc's Rides around mound foloc	pp	ap	—	
1.5					
Riding bike		pp	ap	—	
2 min					
Riding bike LOC(W)	Loc(W) rides off App oc(S)V oc(W)app.sh sh V	pp cc	ap	—	
2.5					
Rides V(S) stops LO'C'S V V OC(S) fol. SV V		cc	ap	—	
3 min					

*State box used to note if a child was upset or crying.

and constructive play, fantasy play of five different kinds, and organised play. Other categories were used to describe the child's social involvement with other children and adults, and hostile acts in which the child was involved, either as perpetrator or recipient, were described in detail by the category system.

After transcription, categories were assigned to each 30 second period: a social involvement category (or possibly categories) was always assigned as these included social and non-social categories, and a type of activity or play category was assigned where appropriate. Times were then allocated to these categorisations. Where there was more than one in a 30 second period, the number of categorisations was divided into 30 seconds to give a rough time estimate. Where the same category continued for some time, the total number of 30 second periods and/or parts of 30 second periods involved were added up.

The social involvement categories were mutually exclusive, whilst the play activities were not; fantasy play might or might not overlap with another type of activity, adult-led organised play might not always be available, and as the time spent in play varied from child to child, there was no predetermined total.

Table 4.1. *Behaviour categories used in the transcription and analysis of the peer interaction*

Types of activity
Inside (I)/Outside (O)
Active·play (ap):
    e.g. slide, climbing frame, riding in cars, kicking balls, running around, inflatable toys
Manipulative and constructive play (mp):
    e.g. sand, water play, modelling, playing cars, weebles (play figures)
Fantasy play (fp):
    fp1: dressing up, police car noises in cars, pretending toys real, etc.
    fp2: domestic, e.g. making tea, families
    fp3: occupational roles, e.g. doctor
    fp4: fantasy roles, e.g. spaceships, monsters, witches, cowboys
    fp5: other
Organised play (op):
    some kind of organised game, e.g. all marching to music
Adult-controlled (AC)
Adult-initiated (AI)
Notes:
I/O to be specified in first 30 seconds and only after if change occurs
AC/AI to be used when adults attempt to get a particular type of activity going rather than for general facilitating of play
fp can be specified and then qualified by Ap and Mp

Social involvement
Predominantly non-social
Solitary activity (sa):
    not near others or if near not interacting or playing in same way or with same objects
Parallel play (pp):
    playing with same objects and doing same thing but not interacting very much, e.g. using sandpit

Social
cc   child-child interaction e.g. playing or talking to another child
ca   child-adult interaction e.g. talking to an adult
ccs   child-children interaction e.g. playing with a group of children
cc(s)a child-child(ren)-adult interaction e.g. involved in a game with other children and an adult
Note: All the social categories imply a reciprocity of interaction

Hostility scoring
Specific hostility (sh) i.e. related to a game or incident
    sh1: property or territory dispute
    sh2: ordering about
    sh3: precedence, e.g. pushing out of way in queue
    sh4: organisation order, e.g. 'You can't do that'
    sh5: judgements, e.g. 'that's not fair'
Harassment (hh) i.e. unprovoked hostility
    hh1: physical, e.g. throwing ball at someone, pushing
    hh2: teasing, interfering

Table 4.1. (cont.)

---

    hh3: insulting, e.g. jeering, shouting abuse
    hh4: pinching, hitting, kicking, chasing
Game harassment (gh) occurring in the course of a game
    gh1, gh2, gh3, gh4 as in harassment above
Notes: Response to hostility from others is coded as h1, h2, h3, h4 as in hh above
Specify if hostility directed towards child (c) or adult (a)
Specific hostility (sh) can be further qualified by h1, h2, h3, h4

However to make the data on play, particularly non-play, more meaningful, social involvement during play and non-play was calculated so that it was possible to have some idea of what a child was doing when he or she was not playing as well as his or her social involvement during different play activities. In this case, only non-overlapping fantasy play was counted as fantasy play and a total of 1200 seconds for each 20 minute period obtained both for time spent in play and non-play and for the social involvement in play and non-play.

Observation of approaches, reactions, approach-avoidance and hostility

Style of interaction with others in the playroom might well be expected to reflect, amongst other things, degree of security or insecurity and confidence in relationships with others. It has been suggested by George & Main (1979) that a child's approaches to others and reactions to the approaches of others during interaction in play reflect the security of the child's attachment to his or her mother. In this study a similar category system to that of George & Main was used, focussing on approaches and reactions as aspects of behaviour which were considered to be of particular importance in children likely to show disturbances in attachment behaviours and social relationships.

George & Main emphasise in particular the approach-avoidance behaviours that a child may show in approaches to others, and the ways in which ambivalence may be shown by the orientation of movement towards others. In particular, they note a peculiar form of approach that they term 'backstepping', where the child walks backwards towards another person, generally an adult. For George & Main this form of approach typifies the extreme ambivalence that the maltreated child may feel towards adults, and it allows the child to walk away from the adult at any moment. Some abused children may become expert in approaching an adult without attracting attention, so that the adult's behaviour can be monitored without harm. Approach-avoidance conflicts may also be expressed in other behaviour showing ambivalence in approach: for example, looking at another person but walking away from them, or walking towards someone whilst looking the other way. The child may change direction during an approach, and walk away. These forms of behaviour are all given prominence in the coding system described here.

The use of a coding system allows a count to be made of certain key behaviours for each child, which can then be compared across individuals. Further, the study of sequencing in behaviour, discussed in the second part of Chapter 8, offers further insight into the social skills and inadequacies of the individual child.

The coding system is outlined below. It aims to provide a core of descriptors of behaviour which are expanded by the use of prefixes and suffixes indicating who is doing what to whom. The data provided by this kind of observation allow the following kinds of question to be answered: Is this child particularly watchful? Compared with his or her peers, does the child turn to look at others for a high or low percentage of the time? Does the child show ambivalence in approaching others? Is the child particularly aggressive? Is the child frequently picked on and harassed by others?

It is also possible, using this system, to look at behaviours in sequence. This second approach, although statistically more complex, allows the consequences of actions to be examined in detail. It can therefore be asked, for example, what happens when a particular child approaches another child. Does he or she receive a warm greeting, or does the other child ignore the approach? In other words, how socially competent is the child? Is the child noticed if he or she approaches an adult? It may well be the case that some abused chidren have learnt to approach unnoticed in order to monitor adult behaviour without attracting attention. If approached, does the child respond in a friendly manner, or does he or she shun contact with others?

The approach and reaction coding system

The approach and reaction coding system, derived in part from George & Main and from Manning *et al.*, was developed and modified for use in the continuous sampling of the behaviour of one target child at a time. The categories used are described below. Table 4.2 summarises the codes and may be useful for reference whilst reading the descriptions of the categories used. These enable the observer to describe the child's movements in relation to others and subsequent interactions, if any, using a limited range of descriptors. Salient actions of staff and other children, where these come into contact with the target child, can also be described. Hence, a continuous flow of specific descriptors is used in order to develop a commentary on the stream of activity in which the target child is involved, allowing sequences of events to be recorded and analysed.

The categories provide: (1) an inventory of gross locomotor activity in relation to others, with particular references to head movements, (2) a measure of frequency of interaction with others, and (3) a measure of frequency of

Table 4.2. *The approach and reaction coding system*

Approaches by others
Staff behaviour
SF   Staff friendly to child
SP   Staff prevents child's behaviour

Other child
OCF   Other child makes a friendly approach
OCH   Other child makes a hostile approach
OCV   Other child speaks (verbalises) to child

Descriptors for the target child
Response to the above approaches
C   Compliance
NC   Non-compliance

Approaches[a]
V   Verbal approach: speaking to someone
HT+   Head-turn towards person
LA   Locomotor approach, directly to other's front
LAI   Indirect locomotor approach, to other's side
LAIE   Extreme indirect locomotor approach, 'backstepping'
CU   Cuddles other child or target child initiates contact

Avoidance[a]
HT−   Head-turn away from other
L−   Locomotion away from other

Approach/avoidance[a]
HT−/L+   Head-turn away but locomotion towards
HT+/L−   Head-turn towards but locomotion away
CD   Change of direction during approach

Hostility[a,b]
PA   Physical attack
RSHV   Reactive specific hostility, verbal
RSHPA   Reactive specific hostility, physical attack
H   Harassment
T   Teasing

[a] The person to whom the behaviour is addressed is coded as S (staff) or CH (child).
[b] The prefix OCH is added if the other child is the initiator of aggression.
All target child codes can be used to describe other children in proximity to the target child in order to build up a detailed picture of the stream of behaviour in which the target child is involved.

Example: The following example is included in order to clarify the use of the codings outlined above. First, a description of the stream of behaviour is given. Secondly, that behavioural stream is shown broken down into codings. Lindy is the target child.
Lindy is playing alone in the wendy house. James approaches her. Lindy looks round and calls 'dinnertime'. She is holding a plate and spooning imaginary food onto it from a saucepan. James snatches the plate from her and throws it on the ground. Lindy yells angrily at James. One of the Nursery Officers calls to them to come and listen to a story. Lindy runs to her.

Table 4.2. (cont.)

OCHLA	Other child approaches Lindy
HT + OCH	Lindy looks round at James
VCH	Lindy speaks to James
OCHH	Other child harassment; James snatches the plate
RSHV	Lindy verbalises angrily to James; reactive specific hostility, as it is clear why she does this
SF	Staff friendly; the Nursery Officer offers a way out
LA + S	Lindy runs directly to the Nursing Officer

physical or verbal aggression produced by, or inflicted upon, the child. Abused children are not all of one type: they have different problems, come from widely differing families and backgrounds, and can be expected to show great diversity of behaviour in interactions with others. The sequential analysis of behaviour afforded by the coding system means that the child's idiosyncracies in approaching others, and reacting to their approaches, can be shown. Hence, the withdrawn child will be expected to make few approaches or verbal initiations to staff or children, and at the same time may make little or no response to the approaches of others. The watchfulness with which some abused children have been credited will be reflected in frequent head-turns towards others, without these being followed through by the child into some form of interaction. The precursors of, and reactions to, aggressive acts can also be seen.

All codings give information about the actor and the recipient of the action. The actor is assumed to be the target child, unless otherwise stated. The recipient is therefore labelled CH (child) or S (staff). Where the actor is not the target child, the behaviour coding is prefixed S (staff) or OCH (other child). using these labels it is possible to give a wide range of descriptions of the behaviour of the child and his or her playmates, as all codings may be applied across all children if necessary. Categories applying specifically to the behaviour of staff and other children are described first. Staff behaviour is restricted to two codes for interaction: SF (staff friendly) and SP (staff preventive).

Codes for others in interaction with target child

Staff approaches and interactions

SF   Staff friendly. All staff speech and actions addressed to the child or children as a group unless SP. For example, 'Are you going to come and paint now?'

SP   Staff preventive. An adult prevents the action of the target child. For example, 'Peter, stop pulling Sarah's hair.'

Other child approaches
These are all addressed to the target child.

> OCHF   Other child, friendly. Any approach directly towards the target child that cannot be interpreted as hostile.
>
> OCHH   Other child, hostile. The nature of this approach is expanded according to the hostility codings below.
>
> OCHV   Other child, verbal. The other child makes some kind of verbalisation towards the target child.

In addition to these codings, all the codings shown below can be used as descriptors of the other child's behaviour, if time allows. The prefix OCH accompanies any such description.

Target child descriptors

Response to above approaches

> C   Compliance. The child complies with a suggestion or request made by a member of staff or another child.
>
> NC   Non-compliance on the child's behalf. The child refuses to do something that has been suggested.

Approaches
All codings for approaches carry the prefix for the person who is approached, i.e. CH or S. Where another child is making the approach, this is labelled OCH.

> V   Verbalisation. This category includes speech of the target child and or other children in contact with him or her. VCH would mean that the target child has addressed another child, and VS would mean that one of the staff is being addressed. OCHV would indicate another child speaking to the target child.
>
> HT+   Head-turn towards. The child looks towards another person.
>
> LA   Locomotor approach, directly to the other's front. The child approaches another person face to face.
>
> LAI   Indirect locomotor approach, to the other's side or back. The child approaches another, but indirectly. This includes approaches to the other's side or back, or sidling up to someone.
>
> LAIE   Extreme indirect approach/rear-'backstepping', to other's front but backwards. George & Main see this type of approach as indicating an approach-avoidance ambivalence felt by the child in approaching the adult. The child 'backsteps' to the adult.

CU   Cuddle. Where the other person makes the move to initiate the cuddle, their marker prefixes the coding. Where the target child makes the approach, the recipient's marker follows the coding. For example, SCU signifies staff cuddles child, and CUS indicates child cuddles staff.

Avoidance

HT−   Head-turn away from the other. This does not include the necessary head-turn which would result when the child sees another compelling activity going on and turns to look. It is a distinct turn away from the other person during an interaction.

L−   Locomotor activity away from the other. As HT− above, it is a rejection of the other's offered interaction, as opposed to a movement towards a new and interesting activity.

Approach/avoidance

Approach/avoidance categories are a combination of an approach, in terms of head-turn or gross body movement, and an avoidance.

HT+/L−   Looking at someone whilst walking away.

HT−/L+   Walking towards someone whilst looking in another direction.

CD   Alternatively, the child may change direction in the course of an approach. Again, this is not simply the product of the child's sudden interest in a new activity; the child approaches the other but then turns away, as if afraid, or unsure whether the other will receive him or her well.

Hostility

Where the origin of an attack is not known (these things can happen very quickly!) a simple coding of PA (physical attack) is used. Where something of the nature of the attack is known, it is categorised as below.

RSHV   Reactive specific hostility, verbal. A child shouts or swears at another for a clear reason, usually in response to harassment which may have been too mild to have been coded as anything more than an approach.

RSHPA   A physical attack, again a reaction to the action of a specific individual.

H   Harassment. The child may prod or poke another child in order to get a reaction, or may upset another's play materials. The activity is clearly malicious and designed to cause distress, and may be directed towards staff as well as other children.

T   Teasing. The child taunts another, but without the physical interference in play involved in harassment.

As attacks, physical or verbal, are of particular interest in abused children, efforts were made to include some brief description of the episode where time allowed.

5   The families

In this chapter we describe the families and their histories. For each family we look at the information available from the casefiles, and the way that they presented themselves in the Family Centre. As the mothers's comments about their children and the behaviour of the children at play and at lunchtime are discussed in detail in Chapters 6–10, these areas are mentioned only briefly here.

Names, dates and specific details that might serve to identify families have been removed or altered in telling each family's story. Such alterations do not, however, substantially affect the veracity of each account. Table 5.1 summarises some of the main characteristics of the families at the time of study.

SUSAN AND SALLY

Background

Susan and Tom had been married some time and Susan had several miscarriages before she had Sally. It was a difficult pregnancy and 27-year-old Susan was sterilised immediately afterwards. After the birth, Susan complained of being depressed and a nursery placement was obtained for Sally. There appear to have been no problems with Sally's behaviour in the nursery at this stage.

When Sally was aged 18 months, Susan took an overdose. A psychiatric social worker became involved with the family and nine months later referred them to the NSPCC. The social worker felt there was a need for professional intervention as both parents complained about Sally's behaviour and their inability to control the child. In addition there was a risk element prevalent in their relationship with Sally. Susan claimed she had lost her temper with Sally and thrown her on a chair. She also said she felt so low and trapped at times that she felt like overdosing and was determined to 'take Sally with me next time'.

The social worker reported that the current problem seemed to revolve around Sally's behaviour. Her parents described her as being violent; scratching, biting and spitting – and as demanding constant attention. She still slept in her parents' room, partly because of inadequate heating in her room but largely because of her demanding behaviour. Susan complained of her inability to cope with Sally, which led to her having negative feelings

56

Table 5.1. *Family characteristics at the time of the study*

Name of child	Age of child (years; months)	Name of mother	Age of mother	Reason for child attending Family Centre	Position of child in family	Mother's marital situation	Head of household's occupation
Sally	4;4	Susan	31	Out of control; at risk	Only child	Married	Unemployed
Kevin	4;5 }[a]	Katherine	31	Held against gas fire; Supervision Order.	Eldest of 3	Married	Hospital porter
Keith	4;2		32	Cigarette burns	Second of 4	Married	Hospital porter
Eddie	3;5	Elsie	22	Multiple injuries; feet injured by scalding in bathwater	Only child	Single mother	Unemployed, was factory worker
William	4;1	Winnie	22	Injured by mother's cohabitee; at risk	Eldest of 2	Cohabiting	Unemployed/pimp
Carl	3;0–4;0 }[a]	Connie	23	Sibling of abused child; 'at risk'	Eldest of 2	Cohabiting	Unemployed
Colin	2;0–3;0		24	Repeated injuries to face	Second of 3	Married	Unemployed
Alan	3;9	Andrea	33	Sibling of abused child	Second of 3	Married	Bus driver
James	4;1	Jenny	20	At risk from mother's violent cohabitee; minor injuries	Elder of 2	Single mother/cohabiting	Porter
Nonny	3;10	Natalie	22	Minor bruises; at risk	Only child	Divorced, living alone	Unemployed
Lindy	3;9	Liz	29	Injuries; ? held against gas fire; mother psychiatric problems	Only child	Separated, living alone	Unemployed

[a]Indicates siblings, studied approximately 12 months apart. Both mothers had another child in the intervening period.

towards the child. Also the family had had severe financial worries: Tom had given up his job to look after Susan and Sally after Susan's overdose and subsequently had not been able to find employment. There appeared to be long-standing marital problems. The nursery placement eased the situation during the day but was not helping Susan in her inability to cope with Sally at other times.

In the Family Centre

Shortly after the family were referred to the NSPCC, Susan and Sally began attending the Family Centre (Sally was then aged 2 years 4 months). There had never been any evidence of physical abuse to Sally but she was certainly subject to much verbal abuse; Susan would scream and shout at her in the Family Centre saying she did not like her and that she was going to put her (Sally's) head down the toilet and pull the chain. Susan would swear at Sally and shout that she was going 'to kill her' and 'swing for her'. On the taxi journeys to and from the Family Centre she would threaten to swap her for one of the babies. Sally for her part would have terrible rages and tantrums, particularly if her mother was trying to change her or feed her. Susan would often have to leave the dining room because of Sally's tantrums, during which she would fling her dinner across the room. If her mother tried to grab hold of her, Sally would go limp and become a dead weight. Sally would scream, pinch, kick, spit and swear and would clench her fists and teeth, contort her face and shake with suppressed anger and frustration.

Susan had been in care for a lot of her childhood and her experience of parenting was limited. She had shown Sally off as a baby but by the time Sally was about 14 months, Susan found herself unable to cope. Susan wanted Sally to be happy and have all the things she had not had as a child, but her limited experience of parenting and a lack of insight meant she had no idea how to tackle discipline. She would stand helpless while Sally had a tantrum, and although she would rage back and threaten to hurt her, she usually ended by locking Sally in a cupboard. She appealed to her husband for sympathy, affection and support, but he appeared to be preoccupied with himself. He suffered from depression, took Valium continually, drank and spent his time in the house reading, effectively cut off from all that was going on around him. Both Susan and Sally found him emotionally withdrawn, quiet and passive. It was difficult to obtain a reaction from him: he did not react even if Sally smacked his face during a tantrum.

The picture that emerges so far contains many elements that have featured in child abuse literature generally: the mother's own poor experience of parenting, the difficult pregnancy and birth, together with depression immediately afterwards, her isolation, and feelings of inadequacy at being unable to cope with the child exacerbated by the bad marital relationship and the particular problem of discipline and control. With the age-related developmental changes in the child, this mother became less able to cope, so much so that she takes an overdose when the child is 18 months old. Unable to distinguish her own needs from those of the child, she threatened to 'take her with me' next time. She blamed the child for the behaviour which she had failed to set consistent guidelines for, and which as a result appeared to be escalating out of her control. Although Susan had never physically abused Sally, she had subjected her to much verbal abuse of a kind that one would have no hesitation in describing as emotional abuse. Sally's response had been to develop what Kempe & Kempe (1978) have described as 'demon' symptons, and the following quotation might aptly be describing Sally's behaviour in the playroom:

. . . they move constantly, unable to stand still or attend more than briefly, and are almost completely incapable of playing acceptably with other children . . . They are very difficult children to manage, not listening to directions, impervious apparantly to disapproval, and forever hitting out at other children. The only attention they seem to try for is negative, and their language is often even more aggressive than their behaviour . . . they must learn how to recognise their feelings, tolerate them and express them verbally.   (pp. 50–1)

At the time of the research, Susan aged 31 and Sally aged 4 years 4 months had been attending the Family Centre for 17 months. Sally still showed many 'demon' symptoms:

> On first meeting the researcher, she mouthed 'fuck off' at her whenever she caught sight of her.
> She would often circle the playroom (particularly on a Monday morning) grinding her teeth and clenching and unclenching her fists.
> She would viciously pinch, and was aggressive to, both staff and children, attacking them without provocation.
> She had low-esteem and if praised would physically recoil, pulling her head back, shutting her eyes, grinding her teeth and clenching her fists.
> She still had the occasional spectacular tantrum.

However, Sally was also a bright, attractive child, who had a sense of humour and could be a lot of fun. She responded particularly well to individual attention from an adult and enjoyed looking at books, helping out and some fantasy play. The nursery staff had pursued a policy of laying down firm guidelines of behaviour for Sally, in an attempt to ensure that she would be able to make the transition from the Family Centre to nursery school. Sally dominated the playroom and was still capable of extreme attention-seeking behaviour, but this was becoming rarer and she had responded well to discipline.

Susan's attendance had been erratic but during the research period she attended regularly. She and Sally now got on well together and Susan no longer shouted and screamed at Sally as she used to. Susan was learning to set guidelines for Sally and felt better able to cope with her. Susan was a friendly, outgoing woman, with a good sense of humour. She got on well with the other mothers but tended to spend much of her time talking to staff in the kitchen and was one of the few mothers who helped out regularly at mealtimes etc. without being asked. Susan was particularly friendly with the oldest nursery nurse, a middle-aged woman who appeared to be a 'mother figure' for her. Susan's relationship with her husband was still poor. He never came into the Family Centre although he did go on one of the day trips. He still appeared to be very withdrawn and wrapped up in his own problems.

Mother and child now enjoyed doing things together and would share jokes, 'muck about' and have a laugh together, and in Susan's words were 'more like sisters'. Susan was obviously very proud of Sally and recounted many anecdotes about her. Sally, for her part, was very attached to her mother and got jealous if she showed too much attention to other children. The Family Centre staff hoped that if Sally could cope successfully with the transition to school, the discipline she would receive there would offset any continuing lack of discipline at home.

ELSIE AND EDDIE

Background

Elsie was a 22-year-old single parent. Before becoming pregnant with Eddie she worked as a packer at a glue factory where her mother also worked. Elsie was the eldest of five children and the only daughter; like her mother and brothers, she had been assessed as educationally subnormal. It was suspected that Elsie herself had been physically abused as a child by her father, a strict disciplinarian, and she appeared still to be frightened of him. Eddie was the result of a casual relationship with a local married man. Neither she nor Eddie had any contact with him. Elsie loved and wanted to have Eddie and she had coped on her own as best she could. Eddie appeared to be much loved by his grandparents and uncles.

Elsie severely physically injured Eddie when he was 20 months old. In addition there were several 'suspicious' minor injuries. At 10 months Eddie had an iron burn on his right arm; Elsie claimed she had left the iron on in the kitchen and that Eddie had pushed past it. At 11 months Elsie reported him to be headbanging and he had a 3 centimetre yellowing bump over his right eye. At 12 months Eddie had a cut and bruise on the left side of his face and Elsie said he had fallen. The day before the most serious incident, Elsie told her health visitor that she had lost her temper with Eddie when he would not stop crying and had hit him across the face; Eddie had bruising to the side of his face. The next day, Eddie was admitted to hospital with scalds to both his feet consistent with his having been placed in a bath of boiling water. Elsie claimed it was an accident and that she had forgotten to put the cold water in. However, she had done nothing abour Eddie's injuries and it was her landlady who had telephoned for an ambulance later in the day when she had seen him. The police had investigated; they found Elsie in need of help and support and referred the case to the NSPCC.

Eddie spent 24 hours in hospital and was then admitted to a residential nursery; Elsie had requested the separation and put him into voluntary care as she found herself homeless. Four days later, following a case conference, it was agreed that Elsie and Eddie could attend the Family Centre. Elsie had found accommodation in a hostel and she saw Eddie two days a week at the Centre. Three months later Elsie was rehoused, and a couple of months after that Eddie returned to live with her – some five months after the scalds incident.

After being seen in hospital, Eddie was referred for psychological assessment as he appeared developmentally delayed and it was suspected that Elsie had not been providing adequate stimulation; at 20 months Eddie did not appear to know his own name and was displaying disturbed behaviour. Tested on the Griffiths Scales at a chronological age of 94.5 weeks, he was found to be functioning at the 78.5 week level with a General Quotient of 83, falling into the dull/normal range of development with scores one standard deviation below the mean. His performance on the individual scales showed some variability, with good performance skills (scale E) influencing the overall score. His performance on the personal–social (scale B) and hearing–speech (scale C) scales was particularly poor – more than two standard deviations below the mean and falling within the retarded range of development. Specifically, on scale B he did not know body parts and could not manage anything on this scale above the 67 week level. On scale C he did not know his own name and his speech was limited to four or five clear words ('nana', 'mama', 'wee wee', 'ta', 'no'); again his functioning was at the 67 week level. Eddie's poor performance on these two scales was considered to be a reflection of his lack of social stimulation due to the limited capabilities of his mother and his impoverished home environment, rather than a reflection of his actual potential. It was recommended that Eddie should have the opportunity to receive daily and intensive nursery school experience in order to increase his social interactions and his level of speech development.

The Family Centre placement provided this opportunity, as well as the opportunity to observe and work on Elsie's parental capabilities. Just over a year later (five months before the research) the educational psychologist reported that Eddie presented as a bright, alert 3-year-old who separated well from the group, and cooperated well in the test situation. On the Stanford Binet Scale, he functioned in the average ability range and there were no significant differences regarding performance and verbal sub-tests. His language development was satisfactory for his age and when aided by an adult he could attend to a task for a considerable time. The two remaining problems were that he appeared to find it difficult to tolerate frustration in play (something we noted in many of the children during our research) and that he had poor manipulative skills, finding it difficult to hold a pencil appropriately and to copy a circle.

In the Family Centre

Elsie was a young woman of low intelligence who appeared withdrawn. She rarely initiated any conversation and tended to reply in monosyllables to any addressed to her. She attended regularly, would sit watching television compulsively in the mothers' room for hours, and always ate a good lunch oblivious to the often dramatic 'custard-throwing' scenes around her. She was accepted by the other mothers but was not a strong personality in the mothers' room. It was difficult to know what she was thinking, and everyone was surprised when she agreed to participate in the research.

Her own family life appeared sad. Her father, a powerful and often violent figure, dominated the rest of the family, who were of low ability like Elsie. He seemed to come and go from the family home, often living with other women. He took money from Elsie regularly: her wages when she was working, then her Supplementary Benefit. She often handed over to him something she was given because 'he needed it', including the meagre furnishings of her flat. Elsie liked going to the 'pub' at lunchtimes, usually sitting with her father and brothers. This was how she met Eddie's father, who seemed to have just used her and then left her to pick up the pieces.

Other people often took advantage of Elsie, and she found herself in awkward situations dangerous to herself and her child. For example, on one occasion, a man whom Elsie did not know turned up at her home, saying that he had been sent by a friend. He refused to leave, and Elsie then had to go out and telephone the police, leaving Eddie asleep upstairs. Later that night a brick was thrown through her window.

Running through Elsie's life was the thread 'I can't cope'; she tried her best but her best was severly limited. Eventually she admitted to the Family Centre staff that she had put Eddie into the bath of boiling water deliberately. During the research she told us that Eddie was terrified of the plug-hole but would not say why: 'I don't like to talk about it.' Eddie had become so frightened of the bath that she could not persuade him to get into it. The staff tackled the problem by allowing Eddie to play with bubbles and a family of ducks in the Family Centre bathroom over a period of two weeks, gradually persuading him to get into the bath with them. Elsie was then given the ducks to take home.

Elsie was short-tempered, and inconsistent in her handling of Eddie, veering between extremes of ignoring his behaviour, even his questions or conversation, completely and getting very angry with him, often inappropriately. She often said she had lashed out at Eddie, but the staff felt this was sometimes attention-seeking behaviour on her part to get them to sit down with her and tell her how well she was doing and to give her suggestions on how to cope with him. Eddie had had few bruises since attending the Family Centre; he never had marks on his face any more and the odd marks on his bottom could have been the usual pre-schoolers' bumps and bruises.

Eddie was a very bright, attractive child, who was a great favourite in the Family Centre. He had a natural talent for mimicry and a terrific sense of humour, which his mother was totally unable to understand and appreciate and often mistook for 'cheek'. He loved to sing, especially to an audience, and the staff had taught him many songs. He generally got on well with the other children in the playroom and was particularly friendly with Kevin. He rarely had tantrums in the Centre any more – generally only as a result of interaction with his mother, who reported he had 'loads' at home.

Eddie could be very demanding of Elsie: he kept on at her, trying to wear her down and to manipulate her. He had tantrums in shops to try and get what he wanted; she often gave in but then on other occasions she would say she had bought what he wanted and that she would give it to him when they got home, when in fact she had not. Eddie got angry and frustrated if he was tricked. There were no behavioural guidelines and he was often smacked for things he should not have been smacked for, although Elsie did not smack him as hard as she said she did. Sometimes she would put him in his room instead so she could watch television in peace, and she also let the 3-year-old play out around the flats on his own.

Eddie did appear to be attached to his mother, although on occasions he seemed wary of her. The staff wondered whether he could still remember the boiling water incident; he was still terrified of taps. He already appeared more capable than his mother. The general feeling was that Elsie had 'done well to keep him this far'. However, as Elsie tended to try and cope by ignoring his behaviour, and she could not control him except by force, it was felt that he might turn the tables on her when he got older and bigger than her. It was rather sadly felt that Eddie might end up in care eventually.

WINNIE AND WILLIAM

Background

Winnie, a 22-year-old single parent, was herself the product of a disturbed family background. Her father had a number of children by various women and the relationship between him and Winnie's mother was difficult, finally ending in separation. Winnie herself became the subject of a care order at 16, having been sexually abused by her father, and she remained in residential care until she was 18. Winnie had been assessed as educationally subnormal but was literate before she left residential care. Then, with one sister and a brother, she moved to London where they became involved in prostitution and a number of criminal offences.

Winnie had been associated in London with at least two violent boyfriends and her initial move to London was supposedly to escape the attentions of a violent boyfriend. When William was aged 1 year 11 months he was admitted to hospital in London, allegedly assaulted by her boyfriend. A Place of Safety Order was taken out but subsequent care proceedings failed.

Winnie and William were the subjects of a case conference when they returned again from London, William then being 3 years 3 months. They had been accepted by the Housing Department as victims of violence, and had been rehoused. Winnie had badly bruised legs but no injuries to William were noted. Whilst in accommodation for homeless families awaiting rehousing, Winnie was observed at times to display aggressive behaviour towards William, but no injuries were noted. There were difficulties with feeding, Winnie becoming desperate and tending to try to forcefeed the child, which had agitated other residents present. Winnie was observed to be immature for her chronological age and to have difficulties in coping with William. She had little idea of how to handle William in any consistent sense and displayed a lack of parental abilities. She was also expecting a second child and there were fears that this might pose new problems.

William had been treated for hyperactivity at a children's day hospital in London. A number of medical assessments pointed to William being a difficult child, with erratic behaviour patterns and retarded speech. His physical development was satisfactory. It was felt that he needed a specialised play provision which could cope with his difficult behaviour; he could be very disruptive in normal nursery settings.

Following the case conference, Winnie and William began attending the Family Centre. Two months later William (aged 3 years 5 months) was assessed by the educational psychologist, who reported that he presented as a bright, alert little boy who cooperated well in the test situation. He was very interested in the various test items and was enthusiastic to attempt the tests presented. He coped with several of the performance items at the 3-year level (for example copying a circle and a vertical line) and passed the picture vocabulary at the 3-year level, but overall he was functioning at the 2-year level. The main reason for this appeared to be his poor language development; he reverted to babbling when excited. A well-developed language programme was recommended to encourage the development of syntax and vocabulary, as well as manipulative toys to aid visuomotor coordination and help in developing his attention to and concentration on the task in hand.

In the Family Centre

At the time of the research the family had been attending the Family Centre for eight months. Winnie was nearly 23, William 4 years 1 month and there was a new baby boy, who was just a few weeks old. Winnie was an immature young woman, who appeared as a young teenager. She was of limited ability and had little sense of humour. She was cold, controlling and dogmatic with William, expecting to be obeyed instantly. She did not really listen to him or talk to him, other than to give him his orders, and would not kiss or cuddle him as she thought he was 'too old for that' and 'a big boy now'. She was almost obsessional in her desire for him to be clean; she could not bear the slightest mess, and she got very angry if she heard him swear. She was trying to be what she thought of as the 'perfect mother', whilst in fact very immature and in need of mothering herself. Winnie often sought out the older women on the staff. Her care of the new baby also reflected her determination to be a 'good mother'; she never left the baby alone and was always feeding and changing him whether he needed it or not, with the result that he was overfed and overdressed. She would also rush to pick the baby up if things got difficult or if she got upset.

The boyfriend was around again; she had left him several times but not very convincingly as she kept sending him her address. She coped well on Social Security payments when he was not around, but when he was there he took over the finances. He was on bail, unemployed and trying to get her to go back 'on the game'. She was adamant that she would not. He had been violent to her in the past, attacking her with an iron bar on one occasion. Winnie was living in the hope that when his case came up in five months time, he would get 'sent down' for a time. William was frightened of him and Winnie tried to keep William out of his way as much as possible so William would not upset him. As a result, William spent a lot of his time at home locked in his room.

William was not frightened of his mother and was always trying to win her approval. However, Winnie set impossibly high standards and William then got frustrated and threw temper tantrums. Since attending the Family Centre there had been no evidence that William was hyperactive. It seemed more likely that his earlier behaviour was a manifestation of the disorganised anxiety, probably exacerbated by being confined to one room, which Kempe & Kempe (1978) have suggested mimics hyperactivity in abused children. William had settled into the playroom and his language had improved considerably. He was a large, well-grown child who was full of energy. He tore around the playroom making lots of noise. He loved 'driving' an imaginary police car or fire-engine, making piercing siren noises. He also enjoyed pretending to be various animals and making the appropriate noises. He preferred active play and still had problems with concentration. His language was often unclear and of an arbitrary nature, and he was a child who often appeared to 'live in a world of his own'.

CONNIE, CARL AND COLIN

Background

The family was referred to the Family Centre by an NSPCC inspector who had become involved when Connie had hit Colin, then aged 15 months, across the face causing minor bruising. The child was admitted voluntarily to hospital and at a case conference Colin was placed on the Child Abuse Register. A day nursery place was obtained for Colin but Connie kept him at home and sent Carl (then aged 27 months) instead.

Connie felt very isolated at home and not supported in the care of the children by Charles, her cohabitee. He was away a lot during the day, occasionally drank heavily and had been violent to her in the past. She appeared to have encouraged the close dependence on her of Colin and Carl, whilst having a low threshold of tolerance. She complained of lack of sleep due to the boys waking early and their constant clinging behaviour. Her ability to cope was further inhibited by painful menstrual periods, although the removal of her IUD had helped this. She had close contact with her own mother but unfortunately this appeared to reinforce undesirable child management – for example, rewarding tantrum behaviour on the part of the boys.

In the Family Centre

Following their referral, Connie and the two boys began attending the Family Centre. Colin had had two face injuries since starting. Once he had two black eyes (notoriously difficult to get accidentally) and Connie claimed she had dropped him on the bus; a week later he had bruising down both cheeks. However, it was made clear to Connie that bruises were not acceptable, and after that she was able to prevent 'accidents' happening.

There was no evidence that Carl had ever been physically abused but he was the more disturbed of the two children. He was highly disturbed when he first started at the Family Centre; when an adult spoke to him or told him off he used to roll his eyes so that only the whites were visible (extreme avoidance behaviour), and he threw terrible tantrums. He would also watch Colin continually, with a 'worried' look on his face, and would try and persuade him away from their mother by telling him to come and play. This protectiveness towards his younger brother was also noted by the educational psychologist when she tested Carl after he had been at the Family Centre a few months. On the Stanford–Binet Scale he was in the above-average ability range, with a chronological age of 2 years 11 months, a mental age of 3 years 3 months and an IQ of 107. She commented that given his difficult background, this was probably a low estimate of Carl's true potential. There appeared to be no problems with language development and overall he was progressing well.

At the time of the first research period Connie was 23, Carl 3, and Colin 2, and they had been attending the family Centre for six months. Much of the time Connie tended to ignore the children and let them do what they liked; then when the situation got out of hand she got angry. She resented her 26-year-old cohabitee leaving her alone with the children. He was unemployed and drank; Connie liked to go out drinking too. She had put the boys into voluntary care – once for a week before attending the Family Centre, twice since, in the space of six weeks – and she appeared to use the children to try and 'get at' her cohabitee. Connie was very self-obsessed and at the beginning of the research was wrapped up in her latest pregnancy. She spent all her time at the Family Centre in the mothers' room, generally talking about herself to whoever would listen, and had as little to do with the two boys as possible.

Carl appeared wary of his mother; he never went to her and would not sit and let her cuddle him. He 'watched' her, particularly if Colin was also in the room. It seemed likely that the experience of seeing his younger brother abused, as well as witnessing violence between his parents, had contributed to Carl's emotional abuse. He was a bright child, who tended to be solitary in the playroom, finding his 'own spot' and playing alone. There was an undernourished air about him; he had lost weight and his younger brother was heavier than him. He also 'wet' himself all the time and usually arrived at the Family Centre with a wet, dirty nappy. Consequently he had bad nappy rash. Both Carl and Colin had gone through a period of viciously biting each other and the other children, but this behaviour appeared to be decreasing.

Connie would talk a lot about how Carl was her favourite – her 'baby'. She had had a miscarriage and then lost a baby aged two and a half months before having Carl. However, this talk tended to be solely in terms of herself and her own needs and had little to do with the actual child. She seemed to have little idea of what Carl was actually like and seriously underestimated his abilities. Nothing could live up to Connie's expectations. During the research she was finally able to persuade her cohabitee to marry her. The wedding day proved to be a total anticlimax, with Connie rushing back from the Registry Office to change into her oldest dress and sink into depression. The new baby turned out to be what she claimed was a 'much-wanted' daughter, but when the researcher admired the 2-month-old baby she was told 'She's evil that one – just look at her', and the child was already showing signs of poor physical caretaking (filthy clothes, smelly nappy, etc.).

The staff were expecting to have to go on working with the family for some time. They were hoping to keep Carl and Colin together until they were both ready for school. They were going to continue to try and give Connie lots of attention to compensate for her feelings of neglect and lack of attention from her husband.

KATHERINE, KEVIN AND KEITH

Background

The Family Centre team became involved with this family when Kevin suffered a burn injury at the age of 23 months. Katherine eventually admitted that she had held Kevin over the gas fire in their flat as she had wanted to teach him a lesson to stop him 'messing with the fire'. She said she did not realise he would be seriously burned. The doctor who examined Kevin estimated that he must have been held down over the fire for at least 30 seconds to have occasioned the wide blistered area over both buttocks. At a case conference the NSPCC assumed primary responsibility for the case and Kevin was made the subject of a Place of Safety Order. After hospitalisation he was sent to a residential nursery. His younger brother Keith, then aged 14 months, was in the care of his maternal grandfather. When the Place of Safety Order expired, both children became subject to Interim Care Orders and were placed in a residential nursery. Katherine was convicted of causing grevious bodily harm to Kevin and made subject of a 2-year Probation Order. She returned to court a couple of months later to contest the custody of her children and was allowed to have the children back, subject to her being placed under a Supervision Order. She and the two children then started attending the Family Centre.

Katherine married Alex in 1975 and there were continual marital problems. Initially there were difficulties in finding accommodation. In addition, Alex suffered from severe attacks of epilepsy and often refused to take his medication, which had caused friction. Katherine had also been unwilling to let Alex take much part in the children's upbringing, as she feared he might have an attack whilst handling them. Her brother Mark had lived with them for long periods (he was staying with them when Kevin was injured) and the siblings appeared to have colluded, with the result that Alex had been shut out and left with no role to play in the family. Alex and Katherine legally separated in October 1978, two weeks after the birth of Keith, but were reconciled in 1979. Their youngest child, Mark, was born in September 1981.

Katherine had swings of mood and was referred to a psychiatrist, who concluded that she was not medically depressed. She had shown little remorse over Kevin's injury, maintaining that she did not know such a serious burn would result, although she did once ask whether Kevin would remember the incident. She visited the children regularly when they were in care and appeared loving, but was sometimes short-tempered with them. On occasions the residential staff observed that she had been drinking; she consistently denied that she had a drink problem.

After the family had been attending the Family Centre for six months, the educational psychologist reported that Kevin had no developmental problems and that his language appeared adequate. At first he had shown an undue dependence on his mother but this lessened. He appeared a more independent, happy little boy, who was responding well in all nursery situations. He showed spontaneous demonstrations of affection to all staff, had good concentration, and ate and played well. There were no tantrums. He could be aggressive with other children if he did not get his own way, but, although at first he used to bite, this behaviour had quickly disappeared.

In the Family Centre

At the time of the first research period the family had been attending the Centre for just over 2 years. Katherine was 31 years old, Kevin 4 years 5 months and Keith just over 2 years 9 months. The staff found Katherine and Kevin something of a paradox: Kevin was 'the most normal child here with the most abnormal mother'. Katherine had a cruel streak, manifested in her liking to tease and frighten her children, which made one uneasy. The nursery staff reported that on occasions she had dressed up as a 'witch', covered her face and crept up behind the children, frightening them. She had held them up in front of a mirror, making faces at them until they cried. Both Kevin and Keith were frightened of mirrors and puppets. Katherine had said to the Nursery Officers that she 'can't frighten Kevin' but that 'it gets to Keith'. She also allowed them to watch horror films on the television and switched on to programmes which she knew had frightened them in the past. Katherine seemed to enjoy teasing the children until they became distressed.

Kevin had not been re-injured; however, Keith had had three minor cigarette burns and a bruised bottom, and baby Mark at 2 months had a cigarette burn on his nose. Kevin did not appear frightened of his mother, although he was occasionally wary of her, depending on her mood. He was progressing well developmentally and appeared a bright, happy little boy, who played well and particularly enjoyed organised games. Katherine mentioned during the first research period that she was worried that the children had inherited epilepsy from their father; to counteract this she was trying to keep them as active as possible and got very upset if she saw them doing anything that reminded her of Alex. Although we were able to get her misconceptions about epilepsy corrected, she still seemed to connect Keith in particular with his father. Kevin was her 'first-born', 'her baby', and seemed in many ways to be her favourite. Keith she thought of as slow and she was very negative towards him. She did not like him clinging around her and on one occasion when the researcher was in the mothers' room, Keith came running up from the playroom with a painting for his mother, only to be told it was 'rubbish'. Keith was becoming more and more aware of this towards the end of the first research period. He would spend most of his time circling the playroom in a toy car, watching the other children, although he would join in and play with Kevin on occasions. However, by the second research period the following year, by which time Kevin had left for school, Keith had become very aggressive in the playroom and appeared an unhappy little boy.

Katherine was a dominant figure in the mothers' room, looking much older than her 31 years. She would indulge in attention-seeking behaviour; when she first started attending the Family Centre she would 'stage' blackouts, collapsing on the floor. On one occasion when she and a nursery nurse were in a taxi with a group of children she flopped dramatically on to the floor, only to get up rather sheepishly when the nursery nurse told her to stop frightening the children. Katherine did not appear to be close friends with any particular mother; when a new mother started attending the Centre they would be the best of friends for two weeks or so, then Katherine would fall out with her. The staff felt Katherine was not as bright as she seemed, and she would cry if any of the staff had words with her. Her brother ('our kid') would feature more in her conversation than her husband, and they appeared to enjoy teasing the children together and were also over-interested in the children's sexuality. The staff reported that Alex was a very pleasant man, who worked hard at his job and was fond of the children, but Katherine appeared to have no time for him.

ANDREA AND ALAN

Background

Alan came to the Family Centre as the younger brother of an abused sibling, Alistair. Alistair, who had left the Family Centre by the time of the study, had suffered soft tissue injury as a result of severe physical chastisement by his father. An older sister was attending primary school. Although Alan occasionally came to the Family Centre with bruises, these were thought to be accidental in origin. Their mother, Andrea, came to the Family Centre for support and guidance in coping with her three children, who she found difficult to discipline. Her difficulty in controlling her children appeared to lead, in turn, to their father's harsh treatment of them. Alan's attendance gave him some time away from his father.

The social worker found Frank, their father, difficult to work with and over-protective. Andrea was rather more amenable to intervention; she was warm and motherly, but confused in her control of the children. Andrea was very reliant on her mother, who lived with them. Frank and Andrea's marriage was clearly in difficulties; Andrea had left for a time, but then come home again and resumed her customary role in holding the family together. The couple were also experiencing problems in their sexual relationship.

In the Family Centre

The staff thought that Alan, as the baby of the family, had been very much fussed over and spoiled by his mother, and controlled by his father. It was felt that Andrea had no control over him at the time he came to the Family Centre. Frank was known to drink heavily, and also took Valium. He appeared to set impossibly high standards for his children. Andrea, in contrast, was very warm towards her children, tolerant, and had a good sense of humour. She would help a great deal around the Centre, unlike most of the other mothers there. With Alan, she appeared loving and affectionate, and they seemed to have a close and secure relationship.

When Alan first arrived at the Family Centre he appeared particularly accident-prone, and would seem to put himself in the way of trouble. Other children would often attack him, but he would stand without crying as they bit or hit him. A burly boy, he would crowd other children into corners, using his weight to intimidate them. This behaviour decreased in frequency with his stay in the Centre, and he became better able to form satisfactory relationships with peers.

One marked aspect of Alan's behaviour in the playroom was his oppositional stand on anything that was said to him: he would automatically refuse to do anything that was suggested. The nursery staff adapted to this, saying, for example rather loudly to each other, 'I'm sure Alan wouldn't want to play with this', whereupon he would promptly come over and set to work on it. A lack of cooperation when he was being lifted caused one Nursery Officer a serious back injury. Jigsaws appeared to be his favourite plaything, and he would spend very long periods in intense concentration upon them. He appeared a capable child, far in advance of the others in the Family Centre. He maintained 'top dog' status through threatening behaviour, both physical and verbal, but could also be warm and affectionate, particularly towards staff.

JENNY AND JAMES

Background

James was registered as at risk of non-accidental injury when he came to the Family Centre. His mother, Jenny, had been in care for most of her life. She had married at 18 and almost immediately split up with her husband; a boyfriend, Bob, moved in soon after. James was born when Jenny was 19. From the beginning, Jenny was worried about her ability to care for and control James, and in particular her ability to control herself when angry with him. At the time James came to the Family Centre, when he was 3, Jenny was afraid that she might injure him. The social worker's assessment, however, was that James was at greater risk of injury from Bob, who was known to drink heavily and who was inclined to be violent.

Shortly before James's fourth birthday, his mother gave birth to a little girl. Within a month Bob smashed up the house and took the baby away, abandoning her, later, at the social services department for homeless families. He also took Jenny's money with him. The house wrecked, Jenny moved with her children into a room in a hotel, where the room was ransacked and the family's clothes stolen. James was very distressed at this time, and had frequent nightmares. In the meantime, Bob moved back into the house, and changed the locks.

During this time the baby became ill with chest trouble, and was admitted to hospital, returning to the hostel a few days later. Jenny found James on the table in their hostel room, and knocked him onto the floor. No marks were found on his body, but James and the baby were both taken into care. A fortnight later James returned to Jenny in the hostel, and immediately wrecked the room.

Around this time Bob asked Jenny to return to him, and promised to obtain treatment for his alcoholism. A mortgage for a new home was discussed, and Jenny began to fantasise about making a good life for them as a family. Six weeks later they all moved together into a flat in a poor area of the city. Jenny said that she felt much better about her relationship with James, and asked the social worker to leave her alone to make a new start. James was said, however, to be unhappy and disturbed, and troubled by thoughts of death. James continued to come to the Family Centre, while Jenny, who was working in a nightclub, ceased to attend regularly.

Two months later Bob injured James, bruising him. The social worker felt that while Jenny was trying hard to take good care of her children, Bob was a dangerous influence on the family. Bob and Jenny's relationship was precarious. Jenny said that she was trying to protect the children from Bob, who was drinking heavily.

A month later Jenny, James, Bob and the baby moved into a new house, described by the social worker as 'immaculate'. Jenny was tremendously proud of it, and very optimistic about the future. Around this time, however, James cut the baby's clothes with scissors, whilst the baby was wearing them, and Jenny, enraged, told him to go to the Family Centre and not come back. Within a month Bob was drinking heavily again, and was felt not to be safe with the baby. Jenny took the children and went to stay at a friend's house.

In the Family Centre

Jenny was felt by the staff to be wrapped up in her own needs and problems to the exclusion of her children's needs. She did not, for example, come to the Family Centre for James's fourth birthday party. Jenny was, however, loving and affectionate to James on some of the rare occasions when she did visit the Centre.

James's attachment to his mother was clearly insecure. He was, by Jenny's account, obsessed by the fear that she might die. This was maintained to some extent by his dislike for Bob, which made his relationship with his mother more important to him.

When James was first observed in the Family Centre, at the time that he was living with his mother in the hotel, he appeared as a lively, attractive child, able to play with the other children. In the course of the six-month research period, however, his behaviour deteriorated dramatically. He would pass through periods of acute disturbance, during which he would engage in tantrums and wild screaming, and would be aggressive to both adults and children. At other times he would show symptoms which in adulthood would be considered depressive, lying immobile or weeping uncontrollably for long periods.

Of all the children in the Family Centre he presented the most severe behaviour problems, and the staff invested a great deal of energy in controlling him, mostly through very affectionate intervention; he was frequently cuddled and cajoled into play. The Matron's feeling was that James needed loving, consistent handling, which he certainly appeared to be receiving from the staff. He required a great deal of coaxing and rewarding, and needed immediate gratification of his needs. He would apply considerable energy to the task of attempting to annoy adults, and bombarded the researcher with a barrage of missiles on one of her visits to the playroom. The general feeling shared by the nursery staff and the researcher was that there was a warm, lively and intelligent child within James, but that he was so severely disturbed that this could not show through most of the time.

NATALIE AND NONNY

Background

Nonny came to the Family Centre half-way through the second period of research. In common with most of the other families in this study, her mother Natalie had an unhappy history: her father had left home when she was 5, there appeared to have been a history of emotional abuse and neglect, and she had spent four years in care in her teens. Natalie married at 17, and Nonny was born two years later. When Nonny was 21 months old, Natalie took her to the local hospital in great distress, saying that she felt like putting her baby's head in a bucket of water. Two months later Natalie was prosecuted for shoplifting, and a month later Nonny was bruised on the head. Nonny was placed on the Child Abuse Register a month later, showing no signs of injury.

A year later Natalie was beaten up by her husband, when he found a love-bite on her neck. As a result, the couple separated. Natalie moved with Nonny to a one-roomed flat, and they began to attend the Family Centre. Natalie was threatening to smother her child. At that time it was noted that there appeared to be a lack of warmth from mother to child.

It was apparent that Natalie was sexually very active, and that Nonny was suffering as a result. Often she would be sent out onto the landing while her mother went to bed with one of a succession of boyfriends; Natalie reported this as a problem, as the neighbours were complaining about her 3-year-old making a noise in the hallway. Natalie split with one boyfriend when he asked her to make Nonny watch them have sex. Natalie was seen by the social worker as a demanding person, in need of attention and approval from everyone. She was prone to misuse of Valium.

A month after Nonny and Natalie came to the Family Centre, Nonny's father, who was from the Middle East, said that he wanted Nonny to go and live with his parents. Nonny, distressed, messed up the flat, and Natalie hit her, leaving no marks. The plan was not carried out. The social worker commented that Nonny seemed to be being used as a means for her parents to score points off each other. Natalie was also presenting many different problems to her social worker and to the Family Centre, and difficulty was noted in indentifying the focus of the case, and appropriate areas for intervention. Natalie was observed to have very high expectations of Nonny.

Two weeks later, Natalie found herself pregnant again, but did not know who the father was. She left her flat and moved in with one of the other Family Centre mothers: both had high hopes of a glamorous life. Natalie was promptly taken to court for the theft of a handbag in a nightclub. She was drinking to excess, and had accumulated a trail of debts. The social worker felt that she needed proper housing, but that this would not be offered to her, given her history. Nonny was exceptionally well dressed and clean.

In the Family Centre

Nonny seemed a particularly attractive, friendly, affectionate little girl, always beautifully turned out. When Natalie spoke to her it was generally to quibble over trivial details of Nonny's behaviour; she never played with her, and appeared enraged by the most winning behaviour on Nonny's part.

Natalie's 'great sexual appetite' was commented on. She would often pick men up for casual encounters and the staff were sure that Nonny was being made to stay in the room while her mother carried on her sexual activities. She probably also saw her mother being beaten up.

Natalie's manner made her disliked by the Family Centre mothers; within a week they were all against her. She acted as though her social worker was her boyfriend, and was jealous of the other mothers with whom he was working.

She would also go into great detail about her supposed ailments, and would tell remarkable tales of these to gain attention, talking one week of her stomach cancer, another of all the abortions she had had. She was an expert on all the tranquilisers available, and would discuss these at great length with the other mothers.

The staff observed that Nonny was exactly like her mother: moody, attention-seeking, with her mother's mannerisms, and would draw attention to herself in the same way. When her mother was around she would run crying for attention, but otherwise this behaviour was not seen. She was a friendly, creative child, demanding, but also able to amuse herself. She formed a friendship with Lindy, and together they would play 'house', cooking pretend meals and feeding the dolls, and engaging in reciprocal role play. Her mother's sexual displays entered into her play, however; she would behave in a sexually very provocative way towards some of the boys, particularly James, lying on him and pressing herself against him in a clearly sexual manner. With the nursery staff, Nonny was generally obedient, helping them to serve out meals.

LIZ AND LINDY

Background

Liz referred herself to Social Services when Lindy was a young baby, as she was depressed and unable to cope alone with her daughter. She was admitted to hospital as a psychiatric inpatient, with symptoms of anxiety and depression, and Lindy was taken into care. As Liz had used over-harsh physical chastisement with Lindy that had resulted in minor injuries, and also had clear difficulties in her relationship with her, mother and daughter came to the Family Centre when Lindy was a toddler, as an alternative to voluntary care.

At 19, Liz had suffered considerably when her parents separated. She and her father had nothing more to do with each other. On one occasion Liz saw him in the street and did not acknowledge him. Liz's mother died fairly soon after the separation, and Liz found herself wishing that her father could have died instead. For some time she harboured morbid thoughts of exhuming her mother.

In the year of her parents' separation Liz married a soldier who was abroad most of the time. They were married for five years, but his style as a 'deadleg' and 'womaniser' caused Liz to leave him. Believing herself infertile, as she had not conceived at any stage in her marriage, she became pregnant almost immediately by a man whom she had been dating for a short while. When Lindy was born he wanted nothing to do with the baby.

Lindy's birth was a difficult one, and she had to remain in intensive care when Liz went home. For months Liz claimed that she believed that Lindy was not her baby, and that her child had been exchanged for another baby in the maternity hospital.

For the next year Liz lived alone with Lindy, occasionally consorting with 'more deadlegs', one of whom bruised Lindy when he had been drinking. Her social worker commented that Liz had a tendency to devalue herself, and to take up with men with whom she had no chance of forming a good, stable relationship. Socially isolated, Liz blamed Lindy for her loneliness, saying that she made her unable to go out and make friends.

When Lindy was $2\frac{1}{2}$ years old she suffered two injuries. Firstly, she was badly bruised by her mother. Two months later she came into contact with a gas fire. Whether the injury was non-accidental was never established. Lindy was removed from home into care. Although medical opinion was on the side of non-accidental injury the charge was not proven, as the arguments for and against NAI were difficult to resolve. For example, Lindy's arms showed none of the bruising that would be expected had she been held forcibly against the fire, and she continued to act normally with her mother. On the other hand her vest and pyjama top had been held up so that her skin was in direct contact with the fire. Medical opinion came down on the side of NAI. Lindy told her foster mother that Liz had burnt her. Liz said that whilst she was inclined to lash out in anger, she could not harm her child in a premeditated manner.

Two months later Lindy returned home to her mother and the Family Centre. The social worker reported finding Liz difficult – a 'classic help-rejecting complainer'. In the next nine months Liz reported mood swings, which were attributed to premenstrual tension (PMT). Her relationship with Lindy appeared to improve. Mealtimes and bedtimes, which had been battle areas for Liz and Lindy, began to ease, with Liz becoming more consistent and loving in her handling of her child. Liz did, however, occasionally lash out and bruise Lindy. It was around this time that the second period of research in the Family Centre began. Liz was at first unwilling to take part, but later changed her mind.

In the Family Centre

The nursery staff of the Family Centre had a rather different view of Liz to that of the social worker. They saw Liz as using PMT as a cover for a cruel attitude towards her child. Liz was overheard, for example, telling her daughter that she would give her back to her foster mother. On another occasion, around Easter, Lindy was not allowed to eat her Easter egg with the other children in punishment for a particularly trivial misdemeanour.

Lindy was thought to take after her mother, showing moodiness and an outspoken nature. Her behaviour was also thought to be pseudo-mature, and protective of her mother. At the same time, however, she did appear reasonably well adjusted. Liz was one of the few mothers who spent lunchtime with her child and, at the time of research, appeared to spend a good deal of time in conversation with Lindy at the meal table.

Overall, the Matron had seen a considerable improvement in Liz during her time in the Family Centre. Having first come to the NSPCC at breaking point, she was now showing signs of change, was giving up talk of Valium and PMT, and was dressing much better. One particular incident had given the Matron hope. Lindy had been attempting to annoy Liz. Liz commented 'She's baiting me and I won't', and then handled an ensuing tantrum very calmly.

Whilst on first impression, Lindy appeared an accident-prone child, running to the staff and crying over trivial incidents, during observation in the playroom she appeared to set herself up as a victim, repeating her mother's pattern, and would invite harm from other children. However, Lindy did spend a lot of time playing with Nonny; Lindy was clearly glad of a playmate, and engaged in comparatively sophisticated reciprocal role play with her. At times Lindy would have tantrums whilst at play, and had an impressive battery of expletives that she would hurl at other children.

A COMPARISON WITH NATIONAL STATISTICS

It is worth while considering the extent to which these children and families are typical of those who were registered with the NSPCC at the time. Creighton (1984) provides a summary of child abuse statistics based on the Registers maintained by the NSPCC Special Units between 1977 and 1982. These units cover approximately 10% of the child population of England and Wales. It is worth noting that the criteria for registration have remained substantially the same as those laid out in Chapter 2, although additional categories have been added. The children studied here had been registered between 1978 and 1982.

The majority of the children whom we studied had suffered moderate injuries of some kind. This was in line with national statistics: 76% was the national figure, while 8 of the 11 children we studied had received injuries of this type. Given the degree of severity of the injuries, however, these children were rather younger than the national average, which is 5 years 10 months for moderate injury. Creighton's figures show that younger children are more prone to the most serious injuries.

The group of children that we studied was unusual in being mainly composed of boys. Boys do generally outnumber girls for any type of abuse, with the exception of sexual abuse. The percentages nationally have tended to be 55% boys to 45% girls, however, so our group differed from the national averages.

With regard to parental status, our group showed an over-representation of single mothers, or mothers in unstable cohabiting relationships. Creighton reports a high incidence of marital discord, affecting more than half of the registered families. Our impression was that discord was a problem for all the married and cohabiting parents in our sample.

Further, while 65% of registered families fell within social classes 4 and 5, all of ours were in these socio-economic brackets. Creighton observed that financial problems were a stress factor for approximately 30% of the registered families. All the families that we saw, however, appeared to be suffering financial problems, and the Family Centre group could be characterised as a relatively financially needy, economically disadvantaged group on comparison with the national figures.

Overall, then, these families shared some common characteristics with the national figures, particularly with regard to severity of injury of the children, but there was an over-representation of parental discord, single parenthood and financial disadvantage. These families had often been offered Family Centre placement as an alternative to residential care for the child, and the families were often in precarious circumstances. The group of children was typical in some respects, but was particularly at risk, living in markedly disadvantaged circumstances.

6   *Lunchtime in the Family Centre*

Lunchtime was an important social occasion in the Family Centre day, all the Family Centre users coming together for lunch at the round tables that were set up in the babies' room. The children came up from the downstairs playroom with their two Nursery Officers to join the babies and the other two Nursery Officers, and the mothers trailed in from the smoky haze of the mothers' room. During their two days a week attendance at the Family Centre, a matter of some 10 hours a week, the only time most of the mothers sat with their children (unless they were very small babies) was at lunchtimes, a period of about half an hour in the middle of the day. A mother might spend all the rest of her time sitting in the mothers' room never venturing near the playroom, but at lunchtimes there was an expectation that she would sit with and look after her child. In addition, lunch was only available to mothers if they sat in the babies' room for it.

The researcher too lunched in the babies' room and soon realised that there was a unique opportunity to observe some mother–child interaction in what was, for this sample, a fairly naturalistic setting. As it was not known how the mothers would react to overt observation in this setting, these observations were carried out after the collection of the other maternal data. Time constraints meant only 10 observations could be recorded: one mother-present observation for each of the five mother–child pairs who were studied in this way and, for contrast, one observation for each of the five children on a mother-absent day when the children were cared for by the nursery staff. The researcher was particularly interested to examine:

> Whether or not a mother did in fact take responsibility for her child's behaviour or whether she tended to defer to the nursery staff present.
>
> Whether she responded to her child's verbal initiations and to the child's behaviour generally.
>
> How she coped with the child's behaviour and what kind of strategies, if any, she used when the child misbehaved or became distressed.

It will be seen that observations recorded offer valuable insights in these areas, which could usefully be focussed on by professionals studying practical parenting skills. It is often felt that children 'play up' more with their parents, and therefore it is interesting to compare a child's behaviour on a mother-present and on a mother-absent day, and to note how well all the children responded to the consistent, firm but kind handling of the nursery staff, who provide an excellent model of child care. Interestingly enough some of the mothers showed similar skills when dealing with someone else's child (see Beatrice with Eddie) – an area that is also surely ripe for exploitation by the skilful professional. In reading the transcripts it should be noted that the numbers refer to the time in minutes from the start of the lunchtime period. Table 6.1 summarises the main features of mealtimes with the mothers present and absent.

SUSAN AND SALLY

Mother present

Susan was generally very helpful on the days she attended the Family Centre, helping the staff to dish out the lunch and to clear up afterwards. On this occasion she made herself responsible for feeding one of the babies, Laura, whose mother was not present. Consequently she entered the babies' room with Laura, 2 minutes after Sally had sat down. She was immediately spotted by Sally who called for Susan to go and sit next to her. Susan responded by getting Sally to move the chairs so that there would be room for her and Laura, Laura sitting in a baby chair between Susan and Sally. They remained seated thus for the next $9\frac{1}{2}$ minutes when Sally ran over to the other table, returned briefly and ended by finishing her lunch on the other table. A likely reason for this move was that Sally resented her mother focussing so much attention on Laura. Susan had mentioned in the maternal interview that on occasions when they had a baby in the house, she and Sally's father had said to Sally that they would keep the baby and send Sally away. Sally was very upset by this, was 'as jealous as heck' and promised to 'be good'. It is clear from examining Susan and Sally's behaviour in the $9\frac{1}{2}$ minutes they were together, that Susan did not fail to respond to Sally's verbalisations, whether they were to her or to Juliette (the Nursery Officer), or to notice Sally's behaviour even though she was feeding Laura. However, she did not appear to connect Sally's attention-seeking behaviour with her feeding of Laura. For example:

Sally	Susan
3.5 Looks at mother feeding Laura Throws knife and fork on floor Looks at mother	
	'Sally, what are you doing?' (Juliette: 'Pick up the one you threw')

Table 6.1. *Summary of the children's behaviour at the lunchtimes observed, with mothers present and mothers absent*

	Starts meal at same table as (a) mother (b) nursery officer	Ends meal at same table as (a) mother (b) nursery officer	Leaves and moves to other table	Runs away into play corner	Cries and becomes distressed	Mother comforts	Mother praises	Lunchtime length (minutes)
(a) Mothers present								
Sally	Yes	No	After 11.5 min	No	No	—	Yes	22.5
Kevin	Yes	No	After 5 min	No	Twice	Once	No	20.5
Eddie	Yes	Yes	No	Yes, 3 times	Yes, for 6.5 min continuously	No	No	16.5
William	Yes	Yes	No	No	No	—	No	21.0
Carl	No	No	No	Once	Once	No	No	14.5
(b) Mothers absent								
Sally	Yes	Yes	No	No	No	—	Yes	16.5
Kevin	Yes	Yes	No	Once	No	—	Yes	15.0
Eddie	Yes	Yes	No	Once	No	—	Yes	17.5
William	Yes	Yes	No	Once	No	—	Yes	21.5
Carl	Yes	Yes	No	No	No	—	Yes	18.0

4.0 Ignores and eats with fingers	
	(Juliette: 'I'll get you one when you pick up the one you threw')
Picks it up	
	'Good girl, Sally'
Juliette hands new fork Grabs salt cellar	
4.5 Tries to put salt on child next to her	
	(Connie [another mother] intervenes, removes salt)
Reaches across for salt and pepper 'I want that'	
	'Sally, don't fight now'
5.0 Reaches again	
	'You don't want that – you got some on – come on stop mucking about'
Looks briefly at Laura 'I want chips'	
	'Finish the ones there first'
5.5 Bangs cutlery	
	'Come on' 'Sally, will you stop the bloody noise' 'Shut your gob' (Juliette: 'When you've finished what you've got, you can have more')

Susan's attempts to control Sally's behaviour verbally were rather peremptory and only partially successful; the calm reasoning of Juliette, the Nursery Officer, was a lot more productive. Susan did, however, use a lot of praise, often repeating the phrase 'good girl'.

When Sally gave Claire a chip, her mother did not fail to notice and respond: 'Did you give her a chip? Good girl!'. She also said to Juliette, 'She's [Sally] being good, she's sharing her chips with her.'

Eventually Sally ran across to the other table where Elizabeth, the Deputy Matron, 'caught her', talked to her and gave her a cuddle. Susan did not, however, 'give up' on Sally; she asked her if she wanted some more chips. Sally returned briefly and then took Elizabeth a chip. Elizabeth thanked and cuddled her and Sally spent the next 7 minutes eating her pudding whilst sitting on Elizabeth's lap. Susan, after making sure Sally was settled, said: 'Sally, are you sitting over there? Good girl, you stay there', and focussed her attention on Laura once more. She only noticed Sally again at the end of the meal, saying 'Sally, what a bloody mess you're in. Don't wipe that [custard] on your clothes'. Sally ignored her and went off to play with the other children in the play corner until a Nursery Officer took them all down to the playroom.

In summary, Susan did attempt to take responsibility for Sally's behaviour and whilst seated at the same table certainly noticed what Sally was saying and doing and responded to it. However, there was no consideration of what Sally's feelings might be or any recognition that her attention-seeking behaviour was anything but naughty. Susan did praise Sally's 'good behaviour' but her verbal commands were mostly not phrased in a way that would make 'human sense' to Sally and she was over-quick to label Sally's behaviour as naughty.

Mother absent

On the day this observation was recorded, Sally sat on the table headed by Elizabeth for the whole 16½ minutes of lunchtime. After half a minute Elizabeth served her, asking her what she wanted, and Sally ate quietly for the next 3 minutes, occasionally looking at the other adults and children on the table. The following conversation then took place:

	Sally	Elizabeth
4.5		'More chips, Sally?'
	'I don't like it' [the beefburger]	
		'Just leave it then'
	'I want some chips'	
		'Push me your dish'
	'I don't like it – I don't want it there' [the beefburger]	
		'I haven't got anywhere else to put it'
5.0	Eats beefburger with fingers, looking around the table	

Elizabeth kept an eye on Sally, asking her later if she wanted some more. Elizabeth had no food left so instructed Sally to go and ask Juliette on the next table, which Sally did on two occasions, returning to eat on Elizabeth's table. When she had finished she took her plate to the hatch and returned to stand by

Elizabeth who asked 'Are you going to be my server?' Sally then carried two puddings, giving one to a baby saying 'There's his pudding' before sitting down with her own. On finishing she pushed her plate across the table to Elizabeth for more and was verbally reprimanded: 'Excuse me, don't throw your dish across the table at me. If you want more, bring it round and ask.' Sally complied and returned to her seat. Later she was allowed to sit next to Elizabeth, and after making an unsuccessful grab at the pudding dish was allowed, after asking, to clean it. She told Elizabeth: 'I want to leave the table', and having received permission, went to the play corner.

On this occasion Sally initiated little conversation, apart from asking Juliette for more food, but responded to all the adult conversation addressed to her. Elizabeth maintained a watchful eye and was quick to respond to Sally's behaviour. When Sally was standing by her she allowed Sally to become involved in serving the meal rather than ordering her to sit down, which proved an effective strategy; she also gave simple, reasoned verbal commands with which Sally was able to comply. Such strategies avoid the straightforward labelling of a child's behaviour as naughty, and reduce any possible conflict in the situation by providing the child with an attractive, comprehensible, alternative strategy.

Sally appeared to be a very attention-seeking child and her mother, whilst responding to Sally's behaviour, often did not perceive its connection with her own behaviour and had only limited success in dealing with it.

KATHERINE AND KEVIN

Mother present

On the occasion when they were observed, Katherine and Kevin spent very little time sitting at the same table. Kevin initially wanted to sit next to his mother but after 5 minutes changed his mind:

	Kevin	*Katherine*
0.5	Runs in, approaches mother already at table saying 'I want to sit next to you'	
		Gives Kevin an exasperated look
	(Keith [younger sibling] approaches: 'I want to sit next to you [mother]') Kevin takes chip	
		(Gillian [Nursery Officer] 'Hey, take Donald [baby; not Katherine's own] his dinner)
	Does so	

1.0	'Gillian, I want to wee' [repeats three times]	Ignores (Gillian: 'All right, go')
	Goes	
1.5	In toilet	
2.0	In toilet	Talking to Gillian, watches Keith eat
2.5	In toilet	Talking to Gillian, watches Keith eat
3.0	Returns. Stands at doorway	
3.5	Approaches table. Whines [no dinner left]	
		(Gillian: 'Get Elizabeth to give you one when she gets in')
	Goes behind cot and screams	'Hey now. Stop it!'
	(Keith falls and cries)	
4.0		Looks at Keith
	Emerges	'Come here! Now sit down'
	'give me a chair' [whines]	'There's a chair there. Now sit down'
	Starts to drag chair	'Where are you going now?'
4.5	'Where can I sit?'	'There, next to Martin' (repeats very emphatically)
		'Get sat down!' Takes chair
		'Put it down there' (bangs it down)
	Looks at mother	
5.0		'Martin' [to baby Martin whom she's now feeding]
	Sits, waits and looks at mother	Mother looks at Kevin
	Moves chair to next table to sit next to Elizabeth. Talks. Gets a dinner. Eats.	

Kevin was eager to sit next to his mother on his first entrance but the only welcome he received was an exasperated look. He told the Nursery Officer not his mother that he wanted 'a wee'. On his return he became upset and his mother finally spoke to him, issuing a series of stern, emphatic verbal commands. Kevin obeyed, but after an exchange of looks decided to move to the next table, where he spent the rest of the meal. There he chatted to the adults and children and was generally well behaved. He did not look at his mother and she only looked at him once, when he shouted to gain Elizabeth's attention:

Kevin	Katherine
18.5 Stands up. Talks to adult. Smiles 'Elizabeth' [shouts] Finger in mouth, laughing	(Adult smiles)
Shows her the mug of water	
19.0 Pours water into plate	
	'Kevin'
	(Elizabeth intervenes to remove mug)
Fingers in pudding bowl	
19.5 Hands in bowl	
	(Adult intervenes)
	Mother goes out with baby Martin
20.0 Gets up from table and goes and jumps on stuffed toy	
	(Sally: 'Can you do this?')
Playing	
20.5 Falls and bangs head. Cries and screams	
	(Adult comforts)
	Mother returns and looks. Puts Martin in cot (Adult explains what has happened)
	'Come here!'
Goes	
	Cuddles and rubs head

Katherine did not actually intervene to stop Kevin from playing with the mug and water, and when she returned to the room to find Kevin in an extremely distressed condition, it was only after one of the adults had explained what had happened that she intervened. Even then, she called Kevin to her rather than approaching him herself, although her 'Come here!' was not unaffectionate.

Katherine too, like Susan, helped in feeding the babies whose mothers were absent, but, on this occasion, appeared to have little time for her own child, Kevin. She was insensitive to his feelings and when she spoke to him it was to issue short, stern commands. On the whole she was happy to 'hand over' responsibility for his behaviour to the nursery staff present, whilst still reserving herself the right to comment on it.

Mother absent

Kevin remained on the same table with Barbara, the Nursery Officer, and four other children for the whole 15 minutes of the lunchtime he was observed when his mother was absent. He fetched his dinner from another table when requested to, as well as fetching and returning salt and vinegar for Barbara, and talked to both adults and childen:

Kevin	Adult (Barbara)
5.5 'Look'	
	'Kevin's finished. He's a good boy. Do you want a bit more?'
Approaches other table with plate. 'Elizabeth'	
	(Elizabeth: 'You have to go to Juliette – I've got no more')
Approaches Juliette 'Juliette can I have some chips and carrots and um pie?'	
	(Juliette gives)
6.0 To Carl: 'I've got another dinner' Sits and eats	
	(Barbara asks Keith if he wants more)
'Elizabeth hasn't got any'	
6.5 Looks at adults as his name is mentioned	
	(Eddie: 'I'm beating you Kevin')
To Eddie: 'I'm going to beat you again' To Barbara: 'All finished' Puts knife and fork down	
	'Very good. Let's put it together with Keith's plate'

However, although Kevin did not change tables for this meal, he did leave the table later in the session but was persuaded to return by Barbara.

	Kevin	*Adult (Barbara)*
9.5	Talks to Eddie	
	Looks at R[a] as he walks to fetch pudding	
		(Elizabeth: 'Here you are Kevin')
	Returns with pudding	
10.0	Sits on chair next to R	
	Walks around	
		'Kevin, Kevin, come to the table please'
	'I don't want any custard' (being served at table)	
		'It doesn't matter, you sit at the table because we haven't finished'
10.5	Looks at others eating pudding	
	Looks at Eddie	
		(Eddie: 'Just cake')
	'Just cake'	
	'Don't want any'	
		'You're still sitting here aren't you'
11.0	Sits, swings legs. Looks at Carl, Eddie, Keith, Barbara. Looks around with hands on head	

Kevin then remained at the table until the children were told they could go and play.

He showed himself on this occasion well able to perform the tasks requested of him by the adults, and when he left the table was persuaded to return without the use of coercion. He did not show signs of distress at any time during the meal and was on the whole well behaved.

Kevin was generally a well-behaved child; his mother appeared unnecessarily stern in her control of his behaviour, impatient of his presence, and insensitive to his feelings.

[a]R = researcher

ELSIE AND EDDIE

Mother present

Eddie approached the table and sat down next to his mother but immediately got up and moved to a position opposite her so that he could sit next to a baby. His mother watched him for a minute then ate her lunch. After 2 minutes he looked at her and away twice, and then neither of them looked at each other until the sixth minute, although Elsie did not speak to him until the seventh minute.

	Eddie	Elsie
6.0	Watches Barbara [Nursery Officer]. Eats	
	To Beatrice [another mother]: 'Don't want any more'. Looks at mother	
		Looks (Beatrice: 'You told me you'd eat it all up')
6.5		(Elizabeth: 'You've got to eat it or you won't be able to go tomorrow [coach trip to the sea]. You have to push the coach up the motorway')
	Laughs	
		Eats
7.0	Talks and grabs beans in tin	
		Looks (Beatrice: 'If you can't eat yours, you can't have them can you mum?') 'No' 'Eat it all up – come on'

Elsie concentrated on eating her lunch and appeared happy to relinquish responsibility for Eddie's behaviour to the nursery staff and other mothers present, only intervening when pushed to. Eddie refused to finish his beans and at 8½ minutes left the table and ran into the play corner to make a den. Beatrice tried to persuade him verbally to return and after a minute Elsie went to fetch him. Eddie cried and immediately ran off again. Elsie sighed and left it to Beatrice to fetch him this time. Eddie struggled and screamed and Elizabeth intervened, taking him on her lap and trying to distract him with talk of the coach trip to the sea the next day. Elsie watched for 2 minutes and then said 'If you can't be a good boy, we're not going', following this by 'I'm going to leave you at home tomorrow and I'm going on me own'. Eddie became even more distressed. Elsie was quite happy to leave Elizabeth to deal with him; she appeared at a loss as to how she could cope with him herself, but Elizabeth handed Eddie over to Elsie. Elsie ate her pudding while Eddie cried and whined, but she intervened when he tried to get away again:

Eddie	Elsie
13.5 Tries to get up	
	'No, don't'
'Yes, yes'	
	'Sit on it properly'. Sits him down
Struggles and cries	'Sit there'
Cries	Eats pudding
14.0 'I want to make a den'	Ignores
	(Elizabeth: 'You can when we finish dinner')
To Elizabeth: 'Kevin's gone' [making den]	
	(Elizabeth: 'Kevin's very silly')
	Looks at Eddie, then Elizabeth and away
14.5 Gets up	
	Looks and goes to get up
Shuffles, looking apprehensive	
	Approaches
'No'. Goes behind curtains	Fetches out and takes back to table and sits on lap
Cries	
Cries	Eats pudding
15.0 Cries	Eats
'Gillian' (twice)	Ignores and eats
15.5 Whines and cries	Eats
16.0 'Kevin's not at the table'	
	(Beatrice: 'He's had his pudding, you haven't')
'Nooooo!'	

	(Elizabeth: 'As soon as mum's finished you can go')
16.5 Goes to play in den with Kevin	Goes into mothers' room

Elsie made no attempt to comfort Eddie or distract him from his distress, steadily eating her pudding with Eddie screaming on her lap. She largely ignored him until forced to cope with him, and even then said little to him and did not appear to know how to tackle his behaviour.

Mother absent

Eddie sat at a table headed by Juliette, a Nursery Officer, for the whole of his lunchtime and only left the table once, near the end of the meal, to run into the play corner. He was fetched back by Juliette, and after asking, was allowed to leave the table.

Eddie	*Adult (Juliette)*
17.0	'You can't have any more yet because not everyone's had some'
Looks around Gets up	
	'Sit down if you want more'
'No'	
	Verbalises
'No' Gets up	
	'You have to ask first before you leave the table. Come back and ask first'
17.5 Goes to stuffed lion	
	Goes to fetch Eddie and Carl back: 'Before we leave the table we ask'
	Brings them back
'Can I leave the table' (repeats)	'Yes, if you sit down and read a book'
Goes	

During the rest of the meal Eddie had sat quietly with Juliette on his left and Kevin on his right. He ate his dinner, occasionally talking or replying to Kevin and looking around the table. Juliette kept an eye on him, giving him second helpings of food and responding to his verbal initiations.

	Eddie	Adult (Juliette)
8.0	Eats	
	'I haven't got mine cut' [pie]	
		'Do you want me to cut it?'
	'No'	
	Tries unsuccessfully to cut it	
	Picks up whole piece of pie and eats	

Eddie ate all his dinner without fuss and only left the table when he had finished his pudding and refused a second helping. Juliette returned him to the table without Eddie becoming distressed, and once he had asked permission he was allowed to leave the table.

Eddie could be a difficult child at mealtimes – refusing to eat, leaving the table etc. – and his mother appeared totally at a loss as to how to deal with his behaviour; she coped by ignoring him as much as possible and made no attempt to comfort him in his distress.

WINNIE AND WILLIAM

Mother present

William sat next to his mother and baby brother for the whole of the lunchtime observed, running to his mother on entering the room:

	William	Winnie
0.5	Runs to mother and smiles at her	
	'I want some pie'	
		'All right'
	Sits down and looks around	
1.0	Looks around	Feeding William's baby brother
	'I want a wee'	
		Ignores
	'I want a wee'	
		(Gillian [Nursery Officer]: 'Why didn't you go before?'
		'Why didn't you go before?'
1.5		'Go then'
	Goes	
2.0	Returns	
		'Did you pull the chain?'

'No'
Sits down and eats

                    'Eat properly'

Eats and whines a bit

2.5   'Stop mithering'
Eats

                    'Pull your chair up to the table'

Eats slowly looking at the other
   children

Winnie initially ignored William's request for 'a wee' until prompted by the response of Gillian, the Nursery Officer at the table. William was then bombarded by a series of commands, which he largely ignored. Most of Winnie's conversation to William during the meal took the form of curt instructions as to how he should or should not eat. William made few verbal initiations; Winnie generally looked at him when he did but did not reply unless they were directly to do with the meal (for example, asking for more). She did not praise him even when, at her request, he fetched the baby's dummy from his cot, and in fact only noticed that William was smiling and looking proud at having done something for her, when it was pointed out by one of the Nursery Officers. Even then, she failed to respond further.

Winnie did, however, retain responsibility for William throughout the meal and William remained at the same table until the end of lunchtime. Winnie seemed preoccupied with the physical welfare and outward behaviour of William and with her control of it; this was apparent in her replies in the maternal interview, too, and she seemed to find it difficult to respond in a more affectionate manner even when William shared his pudding with her:

William   *Winnie*

17.5 Looks around the table to
     Gillian 'I want some more'
     [strawberries]

                    'There is no more now'
                    (Gillian: 'Do you want some
                         more? Elizabeth's got some')

'Yes'
Gets some more

                    (Gillian: 'Share them with
                       mummy, there's a good boy')

18.0 Gives mother a strawberry

                    Looks at William

Looks at mother and baby
   brother

	Talks to Gillian about how William likes tomatoes and strawberries and how expensive they are
18.5 Is allowed to finish off strawberries in dish	
	'I might get you some [strawberries] tomorrow'

Mother absent

William went to sit on a table where Susan, another mother, was dishing up the lunch and remained there for the whole of lunchtime. Gillian, a Nursery Officer, sat at the same table and she and Susan both kept an eye on William, seeing that he ate his lunch and praising him for doing so:

William	*Adults (Susan and Gillian)*
10.5	Susan: 'Do you want more'
'I want some more'	
	'Well finish that then'
Eats	
11.0 To Susan: 'I don't want more'	
	'OK then'
11.5 'That's my big bike', pointing outside, 'I'm a big boy'	
	Gillian: 'You're very good. Do you want another bit of pie?'
	Susan: 'I asked him'

William's verbalisations were rather haphazard and often took the form of general announcements rather than being addressed to anyone in particular. However, he did address comments to the two adults and replied to their questions, and had several 'conversations' with Carl who was sitting on his right:

William	*Carl*
6.5 'I'm going to get run over'	
To Carl: 'I've got some face'	
	Carl: 'I've got some there'
'I've got some face, you've got some there'	
	'Yeah'

7.0   'I've got some wheels'
   'I'm having a taxi'
   [one of the toys outside]

He attempted to leave the table once near the end of the meal but was fetched back by Gillian:

William	Adult
18.5 Stands up, approaches Elizabeth 'I want . . .' [unclear]	
	Elizabeth: 'Good boy'
Goes and sits on stuffed lion	
	Susan: 'William, back at this table'
'No'	
	Gillian goes and gets William by the hand and returns to table
19.0 Looks at Kevin's pudding	
	Gillian: 'Do you want more pudding?'
'No'	
	'Well sit down and wait a while'
Sits 'I want more pudding'	

William had two more helpings of pudding and after being refused a third as there was none left, got up from the table and went to join the other children.

William was a child who often appeared to be in 'a world of his own'; his mother retained strict control over that part of his behaviour which pertained directly to eating and mealtimes but evinced little interest in his verbalisations. There was no evidence of any symmetry between them although they sat together for the whole of the meal, during which William shared his pudding with his mother and fetched the baby's dummy at her request.

CONNIE AND CARL

Mother present

Connie and Carl were the only pair who did not start off having lunch at the same table during the mother–present observation. Connie did not come in until the fourth minute of recording. There were three lunch tables on that particular day; Carl was seated at one; his younger brother Colin at another and Connie elected to sit at the remaining table. Carl looked at his mother as she came in, looked away and did not look at her again. Connie was observed to look at Carl only once, and she did not speak to him. Colin left his table to go to Connie's where she attempted to feed him.

	Carl	Connie
4.0		Enters
	Looks at mother, looks away	
	Verbalises [self]	
		(Elizabeth: 'Do you want a spoon to help you with your peas?')
	Gets spoon and starts pushing at his dinner with it	
4.5	Verbalising to Sally about picture on wall	(Colin approaches Connie at other table)
	Points	
		(Elizabeth: 'Yes, like Worzel Gummidge')
5.0	Licking at spoon full of food	Feeding Colin at other table

Connie was not very successful at feeding Colin; he ran off after a minute and she fetched him back, but he ran off again half a minute later. Connie called him and then left it to the nursery staff to look after him. Carl did not look in her direction whilst this was going on but continued to eat his dinner and talked to Sally and Elizabeth about 'Worzel Gummidge'. Carl and Sally began 'messing around' with their food, sticking their hands in their plates, and Carl then ran off from the table. It was at this point that his mother looked at him briefly; half a minute later she left the room to go and sit in the mothers' room.

	Carl	Connie
8.5	Sticking hands in lunch.	
	Shows, laughs, shakes	Looks. Eats
	Gets up and runs to lion	
9.0	Screams	
		(Elizabeth fetches and sits on chair: 'Sit, it's pudding time')
	'No, I don't want it'	
	Sits, looking towards serving hatch	
	Pushes at table	Leaves for mothers' room

Carl was diverted by pink icecream for pudding and had two helpings, chatting to Sally and Elizabeth again.

Carl	Adult (Elizabeth)/Child (Sally)
12.0 'I want some fruit in mine'	
	Elizabeth: 'You do this time?'
'Yes'	
	Elizabeth: 'Good boy Carl'. Gives fruit
'I've got fruit in mine' Eats	
12.5 'I got fruit'	
	Sally: 'I got fruit'
'And I got fruit'	
13.0 Laughs with Sally	
	Sally: 'Look' (showing arm)
'I'm going in that car' (points outside) 'Can I go in that car?'	
	Sally: 'Eerrh'
13.5 'Let's go in that car' Pushes plate away	
14.0 'Mummy got crack, crack, crack, and the baby in the taxi oh oh oh' Puts hands over face. 'The baby's in the taxi, oh oh, oh'	
14.5 'Ma, ma, ma, sitting down there, The mums in the taxi' Gets up and runs to lion	
	Sally follows

Carl's last verbalisations were to himself; he was often observed talking to himself in the playroom. It was not usually possible to catch what he was saying as on this occasion, and here the meaning was far from clear and it was not possible to determine whether he was in fact referring to his own mother, although this possibility could not be ruled out.

Connie spent a total of only 5 minutes in the room, during a lunchtime that lasted for nearly 15 minutes. She made no attempt to accept responsibility for Carl during this time; she sat on a different table, only looked at him once and did not speak to him at all. Carl looked briefly at Connie once, when she entered the room, and then looked away. His younger brother left his table to go to Connie. She attempted to feed him for a minute but after fetching him back to the table once, she left it to the nursery staff to look after Colin too.

Mother absent

Carl sat at a table where Elizabeth was dishing up the lunch. He ate quietly, talking intermittently to William on his left.

	Carl	Child (William)
4.0	'That's yours'	
		'I know'
	Spoon in one hand, knife in other. Puts spoon down and eats chips with fingers. Looks at adults talking	
4.5	Looks, plays a bit, then looks away	William tries to initiate 'fencing' with cutlery
	Looks at Eddie, looks around	

Elizabeth kept an eye on him, praising him for eating his dinner and asking if he wanted more, and Susan poured him a drink. Carl talked little to any adult, talking either to himself or to William, and looking around the table frequently. He did not leave the table until he had finished his meal.

Carl and Connie manifested little observable interest in each other on the lunchtime sampled and were happy to sit apart. Carl was generally a well-behaved child, who appeared wary of his mother.

SUMMARY

Of the four children who commenced a meal sitting at the same table as their mother, only two, Eddie and William, ended the meal on the same table, and Eddie's presence could hardly be described as voluntary. This was in contrast to their behaviour on the mother-absent days sampled, when all the children remained at the same table for the duration of the meal.

Susan accepted responsibility for Sally's behaviour initially and responded to her, and was the only mother to praise her child during the meal. However, she was absorbed in feeding one of the babies and failed to recognise that Sally's attention-seeking behaviour was probably because of this. She was only partially successful in dealing with Sally's behaviour and Sally eventually moved to another table.

Katherine seemed to find Kevin's presence exasperating on this occasion. He began by wanting to sit next to her but her forbidding look soon prompted him to change tables. She was happy to let the nursery staff assume responsibility for him and it was only their prompting which resulted in her comforting Kevin when he became distressed after banging his head.

Elsie seemed helpless in the face of Eddie's behaviour. She accepted responsibility for it only when prompted and made few attempts to divert him and none at all to comfort him even though he was crying continuously for $6\frac{1}{2}$ minutes.

Winnie accepted responsibility for William and maintained it throughout the meal, subjecting him to a barrage of commands about how he should and should not eat. She ignored his verbalisations unless they were specifically to do with the meal and offered him no praise at all even when he was particularly helpful and fetched a dummy for his brother.

Connie and Carl sat on seperate tables and had no contact throughout the meal. Carl looked briefly at Connie once, when she came in; Connie looked at Carl when he was shouting and then she left the room.

The data from the mother-absent days revealed that on these occasions the children were generally well behaved. The nursery staff responded to their needs and praised their behaviour – in contrast to the mothers who rarely praised their children. Three of the children – Kevin, Eddie and William – ran away from the table briefly, but they were all persuaded to return without becoming distressed. The nursery staff were more effective than the mothers in controlling the children's behaviour: generally they intervened quickly if a child was beginning to misbehave or behave in an attention-seeking manner and tried to provide an acceptable alternative behaviour. They used praise and reward and placed emphasis on the child's good behaviour rather than labelling a child as naughty. They talked and joked with the children and were able to promote good behaviour without causing distress.

It had to be recognised that a mother's behaviour in this setting might not be representative of the way she handled mealtimes at home. The presence of nursery staff meant a mother could avoid taking responsibility for her child and for her child's behaviour precisely because there were other adults there to take over. Also it was possible that in her own home a mother would be more concerned about her child making a mess, refusing to eat the food she had prepared and so on. However, it could be said that the behaviours observed during the lunchtimes discussed here appeared to be typical of those more casually observed by the researcher whilst lunching at the Family Centre in the weeks spent collecting the other data. Moreover, the quality of the mother–child interactions observed accorded very much with the other data collected on the five mother–child pairs.

IMPLICATIONS

The lunchtime setting was one which could clearly be used to advantage in helping the mothers to establish better ways of controlling their children. In some respects, however, the Nursery Officers were in a difficult position; they did not want to move in and take control when the mothers were present, and the modelling that they provided was clearly not enough to get the message through. If, on the other hand, a child became particularly out of control, the mother knew that the Nursery Officers would step in. One of the dangers of having an excellent staff of well-trained professionals is that the mothers continue to be incompetent, as they cannot match up to the models provided. This is not, of course, an argument against having an excellent staff, but one for using the staff in the best possible way to help the mothers take over control of their children.

The ways in which the nursery staff controlled the children could be seen as a set of skills which could be taught to the mothers in, perhaps, a very structured format, with the use of video. The components of these skills included the setting of clear rules and complete consistency in maintaining these rules. This issue is considered more fully in Chapter 10. Some of the mothers clearly undermined their own instructions to their children by laughing at them, at times, when they were naughty. Had the staff seen their role as teachers in a more formal sense, this may well have been particularly beneficial to the mothers, particularly if the mothers had been pressed into spending more of the day caring for their children, perhaps through a reorganisation of the seating and playroom space in the Family Centre.

7   The children at play

When we were first invited into the Family Centre as researchers, it was not known how the parents would react to our presence in the mothers' room or whether they would consent to participate in the research. They were quite happy for us to work with the children, though, and consequently the first piece of research that was carried out was observation of the children at play in the downstairs playroom or outside play area. The children spent the greater part of their day in the Family Centre in one or the other of these two settings, depending on the weather. There were generally two Nursery Officers in attendance but parents very rarely ventured into either play area.

There was an extremely stable nursery population, in terms of attendance, at this time and observations were obtained on five children: Sally, Kevin, Eddie, William and Carl. They were all aged between 3 and 4 years. A total of 2 hours was spent collecting observational data on each child. The details of how these data were collected, the behaviour categories used and their transcription are given in full in Chapter 4 (see particularly Table 4.1). We were interested to see how much time the children spent playing and what they did when they were not playing. We were particularly keen to examine the children's social interactions. From casual observation they appeared to spend a lot of time seeking attention from the two Nursery Officers. Was this in fact so? At their age one would expect them to spend a fair amount of time playing together rather than, for example, being engaged in the parallel play which characterises the play of younger children. From casual observation the children appeared very aggressive, so we also wanted to record acts of hostility: to whom they were directed and whether they were specific in character (for example a fight over a toy) or unprovoked.

In this chapter profiles of each child's behaviour in the playroom are given, in terms of his or her participation in different forms of activity. In the following sections the activity of each of the children is described, and in a final section the frequency of acts of hostility is discussed for each child. Tables 7.1 and 7.2 summarise social involvement in play and types of activity, whilst Fig. 7.1 shows the percentage of time spent in different types of social involvement and play and non-play.

Table 7.1. *Social involvement in play and non-play: grand totals (minutes)*

	Totals	sa[a]	pp	cc	ccs	ca	cca
Sally							
Active play	21.8	3.5	1.6	8.5	2.2	3.8	2.0
Manipulative play	43.2	6.8	10.7	10.1	0.2	13.0	2.2
Organised play	2.0	—	—	—	—	—	2.0
Non-overlapping fantasy play	2.5	—	—	0.7	—	1.6	—
TOTAL PLAY[b]	69.7	10.3	12.3	19.4	2.5	18.4	6.2
NON-PLAY	50.2	4.0	—	11.8	1.9	31.8	0.6
Kevin							
Active play	42.7	12.5	4.7	17.1	4.8	2.1	1.5
Manipulative play	11.7	2.1	6.8	0.5	—	1.9	0.2
Organised play	20.7	—	—	1.5	—	0.5	18.7
Non-overlapping fantasy play	4.4	—	—	0.2	—	1.5	2.6
TOTAL PLAY	79.6	14.7	11.5	19.5	4.8	6.0	22.9
NON-PLAY	40.3	7.1	—	13.3	2.9	13.5	3.4
Eddie							
Active play	44.7	12.5	6.6	13.3	4.7	7.2	—
Manipulative play	10.8	0.2	7.8	0.3	—	1.8	0.5
Organised play	6.7	—	0.4	0.2	—	1.1	5.2
Non-overlapping fantasy play	14.6	1.5	2.0	2.6	1.5	5.7	1.0
TOTAL PLAY	77.0	14.3	16.8	16.4	6.2	15.9	6.7
NON-PLAY	43.0	7.9	—	10.3	2.2	17.8	3.8
William							
Active play	51.6	17.1	7.5	13.0	7.5	2.5	3.8
Manipulative play	5.7	0.4	3.2	1.0	0.1	0.5	0.1
Organised play	3.2	—	—	—	—	—	3.2
Non-overlapping fantasy play	14.0	3.7	—	5.5	1.0	2.2	1.5
TOTAL PLAY	74.7	21.3	10.7	19.7	8.6	5.5	8.7
NON-PLAY	45.2	9.7	—	14.7	3.5	14.7	2.5

Table 7.1 (cont.)

	Totals	sa[a]	pp	cc	ccs	ca	cca
Carl							
Active play	38.4	16.9	10.3	4.7	1.2	4.1	1.0
Manipulative play	37.3	18.7	10.0	3.6	—	4.6	0.2
Organised play	6.5	—	—	—	—	—	6.5
Non-over lapping fantasy play	4.9	3.1	—	0.7	—	0.5	0.5
TOTAL PLAY	87.1	38.8	20.4	9.0	1.2	9.2	8.2
NON-PLAY	32.9	9.4	—	6.9	0.7	13.6	2.2

[a]sa Solitary activity.
  pp Parallel play: the child plays alongside another, but not sharing roles in a game.
  cc Child–child: the child plays with another child.
  ccs Child–children: the child plays with other children.
  ca Child–adult: activity with an adult.
  cca Children–adult(s): activity with a group of children and an adult or adults.
[b]The discrepancies between the sums of the figures in the 'Totals' column and the figure for each child's 'Total play' are due to the rounding up of all the figures to one decimal place.

Table 7.1 shows the degree of social involvement in play and non-play; the first column gives the total amount of time spent in each form of play, and the following columns break this down into the types of social involvement for the child. In Table 7.2 the time spent in each kind of activity – that is active play, manipulative play and organised play – is broken down. Fuller details of the descriptors used for the children's play appear in Chapter 4.

SALLY

Sally was 4 years old when the research was carried out and was due to start school two months later.

Sally spent a total of nearly 70 minutes (out of 120 minutes observed) playing (see Table 7.1). Her preference was for manipulative play – particularly sand and water play, games based on 'sorting' shapes etc. – and nearly two-thirds of her playtime was spent thus. The remaining third was spent mainly in active, physical play – riding a car, running, jumping, climbing – and for 2 minutes she took part in an adult-led, organised game. A total of only just under 4 minutes of fantasy play was recorded, mainly the simpler fantasy plays 1 and 2, which included pretending that toys were real; making the noise of a police siren whilst driving a car was a common example in the Family Centre.

Table 7.2. *Types of activity: grand total for each child (minutes)*

| | Fantasy play[a] | | | | | | | | | | | | | | | Totals[b] | | | Active play | | | Manipulative play | | | Organised play | | |
| | fp1 | | | fp2 | | | fp3 | | | fp4 | | | fp5 | | | | | | | | | | | | | | |
	t^c	f	m	t	f	m	t	f	m	t	f	m	t	f	m	t	f	m	t	f	m	t	f	m	t	f	m
Sally	2.5	4	0.6	0.7	1	0.7	—			0.4	2	0.2	0.1	1	0.1	3.8	8	0.4	21.8	33	0.6	43.2	32	1.3	2.0	1	2.0
Kevin	7.8	16	0.4	—			—			1.1	3	0.3	4.0	1	4.0	13.0	20	0.6	42.7	35	1.2	11.7	10	1.1	20.7	4	5.1
Eddie	7.4	17	0.4	6.7	3	2.2	—			4.2	4	1.0	2.7	2	1.3	21.0	26	0.8	44.7	53	0.8	10.9	9	1.2	7.0	5	1.4
William	12.0	20	0.6	—			—			28.5	38	0.7	2.0	5	0.4	42.5	63	0.6	51.6	72	0.7	5.7	9	0.6	3.2	1	3.2
Carl	4.1	8	0.5	—			—			—			3.2	2	1.6	7.4	10	0.7	38.5	53	0.7	39	36	1.0	6.5	2	3.2

[a] fp1 Dressing up, police car noises in cars, pretending toys are real, etc.
fp2 Domestic, e.g. making tea, families.
fp3 Occupational roles, e.g. doctor.
fp4 Fantasy roles, e.g. spaceships, monsters, witches, cowboys.
fp5 Other.

[b] The discrepancies between the sums of the figures in the columns 'fp1' to 'fp5' and the 'Totals' column are due to the rounding up of all figures to one decimal place.

[c] t Total time spent in the activity within the period of observation.
f Frequency of this form of play, or the number of 'bouts' of this form of play.
m Mean duration of each instance of this form of play, or 'bout length'.

Fig. 7.1. Percentage of total time observed spent (a) in the different types of social involvement and (b) in play and non-play.

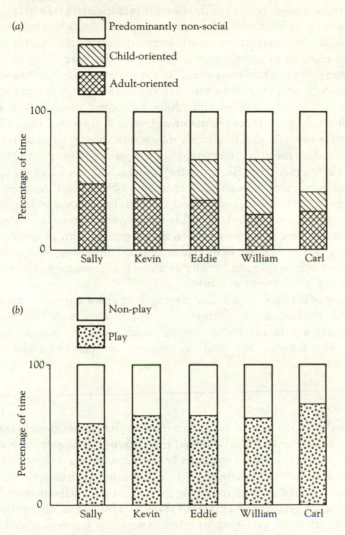

Sally did not persevere with any activity for long but constantly changed activity and moved around the play area. The number of bouts were counted to give a frequency for each activity (see Table 7.2). If we look at the 21.8 minutes of active play, the frequency was 33, giving a mean bout length of 0.6 minutes – although obviously there was a broad range. This meant that in the 2 hours for which Sally was observed, she spent on average just over half a minute on each burst of active play. She tended to spend slightly longer on manipulative play (an average of 1.3 minutes).

Whom did Sally play with? Overall, she spent the most time playing either with one other child or with an adult. About 19 minutes were spent in child–child interaction, slightly more of this being in manipulative than in active play (10.1 minutes compared with 8.5 minutes). Eighteen and a half minutes were spent in child–adult interaction, mostly in manipulative play, and 12½ minutes in parallel play, again mostly manipulative. Of the time spent in solitary activity, roughly two-thirds was spent in manipulative play and one-third in active play. Sally spent very little time in group activities. Of the time spent in group interaction with children and adults, just over 6 minutes were almost equally divided between active, manipulative and organised play. Only 2½ minutes were spent in child–children interaction, nearly all in active play.

What of Sally's social involvement when not playing? She spent 42% of her time not playing (a total of 50.2 minutes), of which 32 minutes were spent in one-to-one interaction with an adult that were not focussed on play. These included requests to be picked up and for cuddles, talking and caretaking. Sally was a very attention-seeking child and the observations here confirmed this. Generally there were two adults in the playroom, with an adult-to-child ratio that was never higher than 1 to 6 and usually lower, so the Nursery Officers were able to respond to Sally's demands for attention. The situation would be slightly different at school.

In the rest of the time she was not playing Sally spent around 12 minutes in child–child interaction, 4 minutes in solitary activity (which included wandering around the playroom looking around), about 2 minutes in child-children interactions and half a minute in child–children–adult(s) interactions.

KEVIN

Kevin was also due to start school in two months and appeared more ready for it. He spent two-thirds of the observed time playing. His preference was for active play, at which he spent around 43 minutes, with an average bout length of 1.2 minutes. He loved driving toy cars, riding bikes, climbing, running, etc. He enjoyed group games and took part in any that were offered, spending 20 minutes in adult-led organised games (Table 7.1). Unlike the other children he persevered with them, averaging 5.1 minutes per bout. He seemed well able to follow rules and if there was a question of winning, Kevin was usually the winner. He spent around 12 minutes in manipulative play and 13 minutes in fantasy play. For some 4 minutes of this non-overlapping he was involved in a 'make it snow' game with an adult using grass seed-heads. Most of the overlapping fantasy play was the police car siren noise of fantasy play 1, made whilst driving a toy car (Table 7.2).

Whom did Kevin play with? Here his preference was for organised games in a child–children–adult(s) interaction, closely followed by active play in a child–child interaction – typically chasing around in convoy in toy cars. Overall whilst engaged in the different types of play, Kevin spent 23 minutes playing with a group of children and adults and 19½ minutes playing with one other child. Around 15 minutes were spent in solitary activity, mostly active play, and 11½ minutes in parallel play, divided between active and manipulative play. Only 6 minutes were spent in child–adult play, which included the fantasy game already mentioned, and about 5 minutes in playing with a group of children, the latter all in active play.

Whilst not playing, Kevin spent the bulk of his time in one-to-one situations either with one other child (13.3 minutes) or with an adult (13.5 minutes). Seven minutes were spent in solitary activity, mostly wandering around the play area, 3½ minutes with a group of children and adults and 3 minutes with a group of children only.

EDDIE

Eddie was nearly 3½ years old at the time of the observations. He spent 77 minutes out of the 120 engaged in play, a good proportion of which was characterised by low social involvement (around 14 minutes of solitary activity and 17 minutes of parallel play: Table 7.1 and Fig. 7.1).

What kind of play did he like? He especially enjoyed rough and tumble and riding around in cars, and spent over half his playtime, some 45 minutes, in active play. Overall he only spent 16 minutes of his time playing with another child and most of this (13 minutes) was whilst engaged in active play. He and Kevin would often race around in the toy cars together. Eddie spent around 11 minutes in manipulative play, mostly in parallel play, and about 7 minutes in organised play, mostly with a group of adults and children.

These times were not continuous. The educational psychologist had already remarked on Eddie's limited concentration span (see Chapter 5) and it could be seen in the play areas that Eddie changed activity frequently (see Table 7.2). Whilst in active play his mean bout length was under a minute; it rose to just over a minute for manipulative play.

Interestingly and unusually for the Family Centre children, Eddie spent quiet a lot of time engaged in fantasy play (Table 7.2), 20 minutes of such play being recorded in all. This included the now familiar police car siren noise, but the bulk of the time was spent in non-overlapping fantasy play and included domestic play (fp2), which was extremely rare in the play areas, and fantasy roles (fp4) (Tables 7.2 and 4.1).

Eddie spent a third of his time not playing. During some of this time he was engaged in one-to-one interactions with an adult (around 18 minutes), but this was not much more than when he was playing (16 minutes). Just over 10 minutes was spent in one-to-one interactions with another child and about 8 minutes on his own, mostly wandering around the play areas.

WILLIAM

William was just over 4 years old and due to start school in two months. It looked as though he too, like Sally, might have some problems adjusting to the school setting.

William spent around 75 minutes out of the 120 playing. His preference was very much for active play; overall he spent about 52 minutes thus and only $5\frac{1}{2}$ minutes in manipulative play. For a further 3 minutes he was engaged in organised play (Table 7.1). William spent much of his time playing alone or in limited contact with the other children or adults: about 21 minutes in solitary activity and $10\frac{1}{2}$ minutes in parallel play. Only about 20 minutes out of the 75 were spent playing with another child and $5\frac{1}{2}$ minutes with an adult, although he did spend $8\frac{1}{2}$ minutes with a group of children and a further $8\frac{1}{2}$ minutes with a group of adults and children.

His mother later remarked that William lived 'in a world of his own' (see Chapter 10), and that appeared to be the case. William gave the impression of being very absorbed in his own play and accompanied it with fantasy play. Forty two and a half minutes of fantasy play were recorded altogether. Mostly his fantasy play was the police car and fire engine sirens of fp1 or the fantasy roles of fp4 (Tables 7.2 and 4.1). As well as pretending to be a monster or a spaceman, William was fond of being animals, particularly a snake. His fantasy play tended to overlap with his active play and he would crawl around the floor or ground hissing 'I'm the snake', or race around in the toy fire engine, his 'siren' blaring.

William was another child with a limited concentration span and his mean times for the different kinds of play, other than organised play, were all well under a minute (Table 7.2). He spent little of his time actually sitting down at a task but tended always to be on the move and involved in very physical play. It appeared that he might find the transition to the school classroom difficult.

CARL

Carl was the youngest of the five children and only just 3 years old when this research was carried out.

He spent a large proportion of his time (around 87 minutes) playing, and divided his time mainly between active play (about 38 minutes) and manipulative play (about 37 minutes). He was a child who made his own spot in the play area; he was especially fond of playing alone with small toy cars on a toy mat in a corner of the playroom. He seemed very vigilant at all times, and if at the mat he would look around the room frequently. Much of his active play involved driving around the play area in a toy car, again watching what was going on and keeping an eye on his younger brother. There were constant breaks and changes in activity, with a mean time of 1 minute for manipulative play and 0.7 minute for active play (Table 7.2).

Most of the time Carl played alone or had minimal contact with the other children or adults. Overall he spent 39 minutes in solitary activity and 20 minutes in parallel play (Table 7.1). Looking at both his play and non-play time, in the 120 minutes Carl spent about 16 minutes involved with one other child, 2 minutes with a group of children and 10 minutes with a group of children and adults. He did not spend very much time in a one-to-one situation with an adult either, although slightly more time when he was not playing than when he was (about 14 minutes and 9 minutes respectively) (Table 7.2).

Carl was a bright child, who played well and often kept up a monologue to himself while he was playing. On one occasion during the observations, he picked up a picture book and started to tell a story about the pictures (fp5). His insecurity appeared to be affecting his social involvement and he tended to play or wander around on his own, making few demands on the nursery staff. However, Carl was only 3 at this time and it was hoped that in the coming year of his attendance at the Family Centre he would begin to participate in play with the other children.

HOSTILITY

The children differed considerably in the extent to which they addressed acts of hostility to other children or adults, or were on the receiving end of hostility from others. Table 7.3 shows the frequency of hostile acts for each of the children.

As can be seen from the table, Sally was the most hostile of the children observed: in the 120 minutes of observation she directed 37 hostile acts towards other children, 31 of these unprovoked, and 6, all unprovoked, towards adults. She was particularly fond of giving vicious pinches. She also attracted the most hostility from other children: a total of 13 acts, 10 of which were unprovoked. Therefore, in the 2 hours for which she was observed, Sally was involved in a total of 50 hostile acts, many of which required the swift intervention of the adults present to prevent blood being drawn. It seemed likely that Sally's hostility would cause problems in the school setting.

Kevin showed no hostility at all towards adults and fairly low levels towards the other children. Out of the 9 acts towards the other children recorded in the 120 minutes, only 3 were unprovoked; of the remaining 6, 2 were specific hostility as a result of a dispute over toy ownership and 4 were in response to unprovoked hostility from another child. Kevin attracted 6 hostile acts from other children, 5 unprovoked and 1 in response to his unprovoked hostility.

Eddie was involved in a total of 30 hostile acts in the 120 minutes. He directed 18 hostile acts towards other children, of which 4 were specific and 14 were unprovoked, and 6 instances of unprovoked hostility were directed at adults. Eddie himself was the target of 6 hostile acts from other children: 1 specific, 3 unprovoked and 2 in response to Eddie's unprovoked hostility.

William directed 14 hostile acts towards other children in the 120 minutes

Table 7.3. *Hostile acts: grand total for each child*

| | Hostility directed by the target child to: | | | | | Hostility to target child from other children | | | |
| | Other children | | | | Adults | | | | |
	Unprovoked hostility	Response to unprovoked hostility from another child	Specific hostility or game harassment	TOTAL	All acts of unprovoked hostility	Unprovoked hostility	Response to unprovoked hostility of target child	Specific hostility or game harassment	TOTAL
Sally									
Number[a]	31	1	5	37	6	10	1	2	13
Mean[b]	5.1	0.2	0.8	6.1	1.0	1.6	0.2	0.3	2.1
Kevin									
Number	3	4	2	9	—	5	1	—	6
Mean	0.5	0.6	0.3	1.5	—	0.8	0.1	—	1.0
Eddie									
Number	14	—	4	18	6	3	2	1	6
Mean	2.3	—	0.7	3.0	1.0	0.5	0.3	0.2	1.0
William									
Number	6	4	4	14	4	5	2	2	9
Mean	1.0	0.7	0.7	2.3[c]	0.7	0.8	0.3	0.3	1.5[c]
Carl									
Number	2	—	4	6	1	2	1	—	3
Mean	0.3	—	0.7	1.0	0.2	0.3	0.2	—	0.5

[a]Number, number of hostile acts over the six observations.
[b]Mean, mean per observation.
[c]The difference of 0.1 is due to rounding up of figures to one decimal place.

of observation: 4 specific, 6 unprovoked and 4 in response to unprovoked hostility from other children. Four hostile acts were addressed to adults. William himself attracted quite a lot of hostility from the other children, being the target of 9 hostile acts, of these, 2 were specific, 5 unprovoked and 2 in response to his own unprovoked hostility.

Carl directed 6 acts of hostility towards other children – 4 specific and 2 unprovoked – and only one unprovoked hostile act towards an adult in the 120 minutes of observation. He was at the receiving end of 2 acts of unprovoked hostility from other children and 1 act in response to his own unprovoked hostility.

There would appear to be some relationship between a child's frequency of hostility to children and hostility to adults: the children who were most aggressive to children, Sally and Eddie, also made the most hostile approaches to adults, whilst the children who were least hostile to other children, Kevin and Carl, were also least hostile to adults. Similarly, there appeared to be a relationship between frequency of hostile acts towards others and the frequency of attack by other children: the more aggressive children attracted more acts of aggression from other children, while Carl, who was rarely hostile, was also rarely attacked.

SUMMARY

In the Family Centre playroom and outside play area the children engaged in free play, with the close involvement and facilitation of the two Nursery Officers present, who also periodically attempted organised games. Several points emerged from the observations of individual children:

1. All the children spent a considerable time not playing, and during this time they all sought more individual adult attention than when playing. This attention took the form of talking, being picked up, being hugged or sometimes caretaking, and appeared to involve the child's emotional needs. This attention-seeking was particularly marked in the case of Sally and one might hypothesise that it stemmed largely from emotional insecurity. A child's experience of inconsistent and inadequate parenting may create emotional needs which get in the way of his or her opportunity to learn.
2. All the children moved constantly; there were breaks and changes in activity whilst playing and changes in their social involvement whilst both playing and not playing. Their concentration span appeared limited, which again had implications for learning and for their ability to maximise learning opportunities.
3. Whether playing or not playing, all the children spent the least amount of time interacting with a group of children. They preferred to interact with either one adult or one other child or to be solitary.

4.   Kevin, who had been described by the staff as the 'most normal child here', spent 26% of his playtime in organised play. Organised play was not always available, but when it was he took advantage of it and persisted with it – in contrast to the other children. Kevin showed himself well able to follow rules, again often in contrast to the other children, and indeed often won games. Organised play involves games with rules, with the expectations of behaviour and social skills these imply, as well as a specific sort of interaction with an adult. The seeds of this more complex social interaction are in the development of consistent and fair two-way exchanges between parent and child, particularly where the parent allows the child some autonomy and control over the interaction. It seemed likely that these abused children had limited experience of such interactions.

5.   Most of the Family Centre fantasy play was fairly simple; police car siren noises whilst driving toy cars was the most common. Eddie and William spent most time of all the children in non-overlapping fantasy play. Eddie enjoyed fantasy roles and also domestic fantasy play, which was rare in the playroom. William particularly liked being an animal – snake, cat, dog, bear, etc. – or other fantasy roles. All five mothers claimed when interviewed that the children used fantasy play at home, but it proved difficult to detemine the nature and occurrence of such play. The mothers were all familiar with the 'police car siren' and Susan and Katherine both described a 'going to the shops' game, which interestingly was a game that the nursery staff generally tried to teach a child when he or she first started attending the Family Centre. However, Elsie showed little awareness of Eddie's fantasy play, and Winnie, whilst aware of William's, gave a very poor description of it. Connie claimed that Carl fantasised all the time: she had in fact been told so by his previous nursery. He was not observed to engage in much fantasy play, However, he often appeared to be engaged in a monologue, which it was not possible to decipher, especially whilst involved in solitary manipulative play (playing with toys cars was a favourite), and it was possible that the observational methods used were not sensitive enough to detect his fantasy play. Fantasy play is an opportunity to test out, explore and rehearse language, roles, specific skills and social situations. The fact that spontaneous domestic fantasy play was almost non-existent in the playroom probably reflected the paucity of many of the children's home lives, with their absence of shared routines and special rituals between parent and child.

6.   Acts of hostility were recorded for all the children, the majority of which appeared to the observer to be unprovoked. Other children were most often the targets, but, with the exception of Kevin,

unprovoked hostility was also directed towards the Nursery Officers. Sally was the most hostile child and she also appeared to receive more hostility from other children. Aggression in abused children has been documented (see Chapter 1).

7.   Sally, Kevin and William were all due to start school in two months. From these observations it appeared that Sally and William would be likely to have problems adjusting to the school setting.

8 Approach, reaction, avoidance and hostility

This chapter discusses the observations made of Colin, Carl, Alan, Keith, James, Nonny and Lindy in 1982. The results of these observations fall into three parts. Firstly, information on the frequency of occurrence of different behaviours will be presented, and the differences between individual children that these illustrate will be discussed. Secondly, the results of sequence analysis are given. This analysis involved the measurement of the outcomes of a range of behaviours. These sequential data will be presented for a small subset of observed behaviours only. Finally, some correlational analyses of the frequency data are outlined.

FREQUENCY DATA

The frequency data are summarised in Table 8.1, which shows the relative frequencies of each of the behaviours measured. These data are presented as percentages; hence, they are not measures of the number of times that a particular behaviour occurred, but of the percentage that this behaviour represents of the total number of behaviours observed for that individual child.

Approaches by others (Table 8.1a)

Staff friendly to other child in close proximity. There was little variation between children in this category.

Staff friendly approach. This formed the greatest percentage of the behaviours experienced by the child for all children except Nonny, with a range from 13.8 to 25.8% of interactions. Carl and James seemed to experience the greatest proportion of these approaches, and in both cases it is quite likely that the staff were using these friendly approaches to prevent hostile behaviour between children for a considerable proportion of the time. Nonny showed the lowest percentage of staff friendly approaches (13.8%); for her, talking to and playing with other children accounted for a rather higher percentage of her activity.

114

Staff preventive action. Nonny and Alan were the two children who experienced the highest percentage of this type of approach, but it is notable, and a credit to the staff, that the staff were able to maintain a warm, peaceful, yet lively environment without needing to use clearly 'disciplinary' means of control. Preventive action by the staff formed a very small percentage of the behaviour in which the child was involved.

Staff cuddles child. James had the highest proportion of staff cuddles; again, some of these were examples of gentle control on the part of staff. It is perhaps worthy of note that Lindy was not cuddled at all during any of the observation periods.

Other child friendly approach. This category shows a frequency of occurrence which is uniformly low for all children. It is probable that such approaches were in fact more frequent, but that they were lost during observation as more salient behaviour of the target child was attended to.

Other child cuddles. This behaviour was only recorded for Alan. Again, as with the previous category, it is probable that some occurrences were not noted at the time.

Other child speaks to child. This category showed considerable differences between children. Hence, for example, only 1.6% of the behaviours in which Alan was involved were of this kind, compared with 14.6 for Lindy. Carl and James also experienced a comparatively low percentage of behaviour of this kind. This measure seems to discriminate between those children who are frequently approached by others and those who are not. For Colin, being spoken to by other children formed a comparatively large proportion of his experience; his brother Carl in particular would often address him. For Nonny and Lindy, the figures complement one another; these two children played together a lot, and the percentages reflect this.

Reactions to others

Compliance and non-compliance. The children's responses to the behaviour of others included in any of the categories above was coded, where appropriate, for compliance or non-compliance. These categories again showed comparatively little variation between children, with the exception of Carl who showed a rather higher percentage of non-compliance compared with the other children.

Table 8.1.(a) *Approach and avoidance of others expressed as a percentage of total behaviours of this kind*

	Colin	Carl	Alan	Keith	James	Nonny	Lindy
Approaches by others							
Staff friendly to other child in close proximity	3.2	4.3	3.9	4.0	3.8	4.7	1.8
Staff friendly approach	15.5	25.8	17.5	16.8	22.3	13.8	17.6
Staff preventative action	0.2	0.8	1.9	0.2	2.5	2.7	1.0
Staff cuddles child	0.8	0.8	0.6	0.8	1.1	0.6	0
Other child friendly approach	0.6	1.0	0.3	1.2	0.2	0.7	0.8
Other child cuddles	—	—	1.3	—	—	—	—
Other child speaks to child	10.1	5.2	1.6	4.8	5.3	11.5	14.6
Reactions to others							
Compliance	5.0	5.7	0.3	5.0	3.1	3.5	3.9
Non-compliance	0.2	1.7	0.3	0.4	0.2	0.5	—
Approach and avoidance of others							
Behaviour directed towards staff							
Head-turn towards staff	13.0	12.3	8.4	15.2	7.4	7.1	13.1
Locomotor approach to staff	3.4	2.6	5.8	6.2	5.3	2.7	1.8
Indirect locomotor approach to staff, to side	3.2	1.5	3.9	2.6	1.9	2.2	1.2
Extreme indirect locomotor approach to staff, backstepping	—	0.1	0.3	0.4	0.2	—	—
Head-turn away from staff	0.2	0.4	0.3	1.2	1.3	0.1	—
Locomotion away from staff	0.8	0.7	1.3	3.4	1.1	1.2	0.2
Approach/avoidance of staff	0.2	0.1	0.3	0.2	0.8	—	—
Change of direction during approach	1.1	—	1.9	1.2	—	0.5	0.4
Total proportion of observations indicating ambivalence towards staff/negative behaviour (indirect to change of direction)	5.5	2.8	8.0	9.0	5.5	4.0	1.8

Behaviour directed towards other children

Head-turn towards child	8.0	5.8	3.8	5.8	5.5	4.7	12.0
Locomotor approach	1.4	4.3	3.1	3.0	2.6	3.1	3.6
Indirect locomotor approach	—	0.1	—	0.2	0.6	0.1	—
Head-turn away from child	0.4	—	—	0.6	0.6	0.4	—
Locomotion away from child	0.2	1.2	0.1	0.8	—	0.3	—
Approach/avoidance of child	—	0.1	—	0.2	—	—	—
Change of direction during approach	0.2	0.3	—	0.6	—	0.3	0.4
Total proportion of observations indicating ambivalence in approaching other children (indirect to change of direction)	0.8	1.7	1.0	2.4	1.2	1.1	0.4
Other approaches							
Staff							
Speaking to staff	10.4	9.3	17.0	12.0	13.0	12.4	10.3
Cuddles staff	0.2	0.6	—	1.2	0.3	0.3	0.8
Child							
Speaking to child	14.1	15.1	8.2	3.4	8.8	6.7	8.4
Cuddles child	1.0	0.1	0.4	0.4	0.3	0.1	—
Other child							
Locomotor approaches	2.3	2.7	1.5	2.2	4.2	2.2	0.4
Locomotor departures (avoidance)	0.2	0.6	0.2	—	0.6	—	—

Approach and avoidance of others (Table 8.1a)

Behaviour directed towards staff

Head-turn towards staff. Children varied considerably in the percentage of behaviour for which this category accounted. Colin, Carl, Keith and Lindy spent the greatest proportion of time looking towards staff members. For Keith, the percentage was particularly high. This might be taken to indicate that these were the children who were most watchful, and, indeed, it appeared to be felt amongst the staff that Colin and Carl were watchful children. To the outside observer, however, Keith also appeared watchful, and he could be seen to adopt a mode of play that allowed for this. He would find a bicycle or tricycle and ride round and round the playroom or around the outdoor play area and would spend a great deal of this time watching others, rather than simply riding for the enjoyment of it.

Locomotor approaches to staff. There was some variability between children as regards this category of behaviour. Keith, who spent the highest percentage of time watching the staff, also spent the highest percentage in approaching them. Lindy, on the other hand, who watched a considerable amount, approached comparatively infrequently. It is the behaviours following these approaches that are, however, of particular interest in highlighting differences between children, and these will be discussed in the section on sequences of behaviour (p. 123).

Indirect approach to staff. This category of behaviour involved a less direct approach to a staff member, with the child coming up to the staff member's side. Colin and Alan showed the highest percentage of such approaches, but the percentages do not vary greatly between children, the range being 1.2–3.9%.

Extreme indirect approach to staff. This kind of approach has been stressed by George and Main (1979) as a peculiarity of abused children, but was rarely seen amongst this group. There are various possible explanations for this. One is that the observer missed some instances, but it is perhaps more likely, however, that the children in the Family Centre had such a good relationship with each of the staff members in the small nursery that they did not feel the fear that would result in this kind of approach. It would have been valuable to observe these kinds of approaches in relation to the mothers.

Head-turn away from staff. This was a comparatively little-used category, showing little variation between children, although Keith and James showed the highest percentage of this form of avoidance.

Locomotion away from staff. This was seen to account for a varied percentage of the behaviour of the children. Keith showed the highest percentage of this kind of avoidance, and Lindy, the lowest. It was more frequently observed than the approach-avoidance behaviours that indicate most clearly ambivalence or a lack of confidence in approaching others.

Approach-avoidance of staff. This behaviour was not recorded at all for either of the girls. All the boys showed at least one instance of it, James having the highest percentage. It is important to note, however, that this form of behaviour was very rare, and would not, therefore, be a particularly useful index of behaviour in the short-term assessment of children if used alone.

Change of direction during approach. This category accounted for a slightly larger percentage of the behaviour seen for some children than did approach-avoidance of staff. As the following section on sequences of behaviour will show, this particular form of behaviour was of considerable importance in Colin's case.

Total percentage of observations showing ambivalence. While the approach or avoidance of staff was comparatively rare, the summary of these data allow a comparison between children to be made. The scores shown in Table 8.1(*a*) are totals made up of the percentages for indirect and extreme indirect approaches, head-turns away from staff, walking away from staff, approach-avoidance and change of direction. All of these behaviours, while rare, indicate that certain children show a particularly high percentage of these forms of behaviour. It was notable that Keith, who had been observed to be very watchful of staff, was also ambivalent in his approaches to them and showed some avoidance. Alan was also inclined to be avoidant, which agreed with staff impressions that he was a difficult child. The summary figures tend to show that ambivalence in approaches to adults might be one useful area of study regarding abused children, alerting the observer, as it does, to behaviour that may well not have been noticed by staff members actively involved with the children – behaviour which may indicate difficulty in relating successfully to adults.

Behaviour directed towards other children

Head-turn towards child. Colin in particular showed a high percentage of this kind of behaviour. In addition to being watchful of staff, he was also watchful of other children. Overall, 25% of his behaviour was composed of looking towards staff or other children. Keith, who had been particularly watchful of adults, did not show a particularly high percentage of head-turns towards other children. Lindy, however, showed a higher percentage of head-turns towards children. For her, 21% of observed behaviours involved looking at either staff or other children. This contrasts with the behaviour of James, who spent a very small percentage of time looking at others (11% in all). He showed the lowest percentage of head-turns towards others. It is possible that there is some optimal level of monitoring of the environment for the child at play, in order for him or her to be sensitive to the things that adults and other children are doing and to be able to join in. Within a small sample it is not possible to assess what this range might be, nor what might be seen in a 'normal' nursery group. Keith, however, seemed to spend so much time looking that he did not spend enough time in contact with others. James, on the other hand, was a difficult child in the nursery group and, it could be argued, not sufficiently aware of the good things going on around him.

Locomotor approaches to other children. The percentages for this category were similar for all the children with the exception of Lindy, for whom approaches to other children were less frequent.

Indirect locomotor approaches. These were very rarely observed.

Head-turn away from child. This was also observed very infrequently.

Locomotion away from child. This was rare too, and not all children were observed to engage in this behaviour.

Approach-avoidance and change of direction. These categories were also seen very infrequently. Overall, ambivalent approaches towards or avoidance of other children were very rarely observed. Keith showed the highest composite score for avoidance of other children, at 2.4% of all behaviour observed.

Other approaches

Speaking to staff. This category showed some variation between children. For James, speaking to staff accounted for a comparatively high percentage of his behaviours, and for Nonny, comparatively few.

Cuddles staff. All the children had low percentages for this category, so that any comments made must take account of this. Lindy had at least one cuddle with a staff member during observation, and it was one that she had initiated. James, on the other hand, did not initiate any cuddles with staff members, although he showed the highest percentage of cuddles initiated by staff. This may mean either that he did not particularly want to be cuddled, or that staff sought him out sufficiently frequently that he did not feel a need to initiate a cuddle himself. It is possible that the staff felt a particular need to cuddle him because of, perhaps, his attractiveness, or in order to compensate for his unhappy background.

Speaking to other child. This category showed wide variation between children. Keith had the lowest percentage, only 3.4% of his observed behaviour taking this form. Lindy and Nonny, on the other hand, showed far higher percentages: around 14% and 15% respectively. This reflects the considerable amount of time that they spent in playing together.

Cuddles child. Children cuddling each other was noted comparatively rarely.

Other child approach and avoidance. This behaviour was noted, but only rarely. This, again, may well not reflect the true state of affairs, but rather that the observer was so engrossed in the behaviour of the target child that these other behaviours were not adequately recorded.

Hostile approaches and reactions (Table 8.1b)

Staff-directed hostility

A range of behaviours was recorded under this heading, as it was considered important to assess the extent to which individual children expressed hostility to staff members. It turned out, however, that these forms of behaviour were very rarely seen. Composite scores for the total percentage of behaviours involving hostility to staff showed that Carl and Keith were not observed to engage in any hostility towards staff, and Colin, Nonny and Lindy, on only one or two occasions each. Alan showed the highest percentage, with 2.2% of his behaviours taking this form. James was second, at 1.5%.

Whilst these figures are of some interest for academic purposes, these incidents were so rare that, for the professional requiring information on hostility to staff, it would probably be better simply to ask staff for an account of any recent attacks or hostility that children have shown towards them. This would allow for analysis of antecedents and subsequent behaviour. While hostile acts towards staff are potentially important behaviours to observe, they may occur so rarely that they cannot be adequately covered within a short period of observation. A record of total number of instances of hostility to staff would probably be adequate.

Child-directed hostility
The percentages for individual categories of hostility towards children were also low. The total scores, however, do show some variability between

Table 8.1.(b) Hostile approaches and reactions expressed as a percentage of total behaviours of this kind

	Colin	Carl	Alan	Keith	James	Nonny	Lindy
Staff-directed							
Reactive specific physical attack	0.2	—	—	—	0.4	0.1	—
Reactive specific verbal hostility	—	—	0.3	—	—	—	0.4
Harassment	—	—	1.9	—	1.1	0.3	—
Physical attack	—	—	—	—	—	—	—
Child-directed							
Reactive specific physical attack	0.2	0.1	—	—	—	0.5	0.4
Reactive specific verbal hostility	0.2	1.0	1.0	0.4	1.1	1.5	0.2
Harassment	—	—	1.3	—	1.1	0.5	0.2
Teasing	—	—	1.0	0.2	—	0.1	—
Physical attack	—	—	1.3	0.2	0.8	0.2	1.6
Other child: hostile approaches and reactions							
Reactive specific physical attack	0.2	0.1	—	—	—	0.1	0.2
Reactive specific verbal hostility	—	—	0.3	0.2	—	0.9	0.4
Harassment	—	1.1	—	0.4	1.0	0.6	—
Physical attack	—	0.3	—	0.2	0.2	0.1	0.8
Total hostility to staff	0.2	—	2.2	—	1.5	0.4	0.4
Total hostility to children	0.4	1.1	4.6	0.8	3.0	2.8	2.4
Total hostility to others	0.6	1.1	6.8	0.8	4.5	3.2	2.8
Total hostility from others	0.2	1.5	0.3	0.8	1.2	1.7	1.6

children. Alan emerged with the highest percentage for this group of behaviours, and James was second. Again, a record of the total number of aggressive acts towards other children might well be adequate for professional use in the Family Centre or similar setting.

Overall hostility

From the categories set out in the outline of behaviour codings, totals were computed for the percentage of hostility to others and for the frequency of hostile behaviours towards the child. These figures showed that Alan was the child with the highest percentage of hostile behaviours to others, (6.8%), with James next (4.5%). Nonny had the third-highest percentage of aggressive behaviours (3.2%). Colin and Keith were notable for the very low percentages of hostile behaviours to others, Keith showing no hostility to staff at all during the period of observation.

To what extent was hostility provoked by others? Alan did not appear to be troubled by the hostile acts of others; he was very rarely approached in this way by other children. The only other child showing such a low percentage of hostile approaches from others was Colin. Looking back to the figures for friendly approaches by other children, Alan was one of the most rarely approached children. Given his apparently unprovoked aggressive attacks, this is hardly surprising. These kinds of results indicate the potential value of examining sequences of behaviour, rather than simple frequencies. It is to this kind of analysis that we now turn.

SEQUENCES OF BEHAVIOUR

An alternative way of looking at the observational data obtained is to make a sequential analysis of behavioural units, in order to discover the most frequent outcomes of a particular act for the child. Using the sequence analysis package, ODLAG, available on the computer in the Department of Psychology at the University of Manchester, frequency of outcomes of a selection of the behaviours studied were calculated. Where behaviours were observed comparatively infrequently, namely the aggression and hostility categories, this form of analysis is not particularly helpful. Where behaviours were comparatively frequent, however, the differences seen between individual children in the outcomes of behaviour are extremely interesting and offer information not provided by the percentage data presented above.

To provide a complete matrix of all behaviours against all other behaviours was beyond the scope of the computer package available. Rather, matrices of a small subset of behaviours were prepared. The data for these analyses are given in Tables 8.2 to 8.8. These tables show, for each individual child, the behaviour most frequently seen to follow a particular behaviour of interest, the number of times this outcome was seen, the total number of observations of the initial behaviour of interest, and the percentage of times that a particular outcome was associated with the initial behaviour of interest. For example, as can be seen in Table 8.2, Carl was observed to turn his head towards a staff member 85 times. Twenty-five of these occurrences (29%) were followed by a staff friendly utterance. Seventeen (20%) were followed by Carl speaking to a staff member.

In general, only the two most frequent outcomes have been reported. Where there are ties in the ranking of outcomes, these have been included in the tables.

Behaviour directed towards staff

Behaviour following a head-turn towards a staff member (Table 8.2). This category of behaviour had been seen as a potential indicator of watchfulness on the child's behalf, and is frequently noted in abused children. For Colin, this behaviour was followed by three other behaviours with equal frequency: by staff friendly, speaking to staff, or with another head-turn to a staff member. Lindy also showed this kind of patterning of behaviour. Carl, Keith, James and Nonny all showed a similar pattern of outcomes to one another: either speaking to staff or being on the receiving end of a friendly comment from a staff member. These staff friendly responses were, it should be remembered, a response only to a look from the child, and the high number of staff friendly responses again testifies to the high quality and alertness of the staff. Alan, however, stands out as an exception. Unlike the other children, staff friendly responses rarely followed a head-turn. Instead, Alan would either sidle up to a staff member or initiate conversation. It would appear that Alan's head-turns were not responded to in the same way as those of the other children in the nursery, perhaps because of his hostility to other children.

Behaviour following a direct approach to a staff member (Table 8.3). Following this kind of approach, almost all the children went on to conversation with staff, in the form of either speaking to staff or a staff friendly response. Colin, however, did not conform to this pattern. This rather timid child would speak to staff or change direction during approach, indicating an approach-avoidance conflict. There are noteworthy differences between the other children in the percentage of staff friendly responses that followed on from an approach. James had 37% of his approaches responded to by a staff friendly comment. Lindy, who rarely approached staff directly, also had a very high percentage of staff friendly responses.

Behaviour following an indirect approach to a staff member (Table 8.4). As the table shows, there was a considerable range of behaviours that followed this

Table 8.2. *Behaviour following a head-turn towards a staff member*

Name	Behaviour following	Total	No. of observations of criterion	As %
Colin	Staff friendly	8	61	13
	Head-turn towards staff	8		13
	Speaking to staff	8		13
Carl	Staff friendly	25	85	29
	Speaking to staff	17		20
Alan	Indirect approach to staff	4	26	15
	Speaking to staff	4		15
Keith	Staff friendly	13	71	18
	Head-turn towards staff	12		17
James	Speaking to staff	11	38	29
	Staff friendly	10		26
Nonny	Speaking to staff	7	55	13
	Staff friendly	5		9
Lindy	Staff friendly	13	64	20
	Head-turn towards staff	10		16
	Speaking to staff	10		16

Table 8.3. *Behaviour following a direct approach to a staff member*

Name	Behaviour following	Total	No. of observations of criterion	As %
Colin	Speaking to staff	4	16	25
	Change of direction	4		25
Carl	Staff friendly	6	18	33
	Speaking to staff	6		33
Alan	Speaking to staff	5	18	28
	Staff friendly	4		22
Keith	Staff friendly	7	31	23
	Speaking to staff	7		23
James	Staff friendly	10	27	37
	Speaking to staff	6		22
Nonny	Staff friendly	6	19	32
	Speaking to staff	4		21
Lindy	Staff friendly	6	9	33

Table 8.4. *Behaviour following an indirect approach to a staff member*

Name	Behaviour following	Total	No. of observations of criterion	As %
Colin	Staff friendly	3	15	20
	Indirect approach to staff	3		20
Carl	Speaking to staff	3	11	27
Alan	Staff friendly	4	12	33
	Speaking to staff	3		25
Keith	Indirect approach to staff	3	13	23
	Speaking to staff	3		23
James	Staff friendly	2	10	20
	Direct approach to staff	2		20
Nonny	Staff friendly	6	17	35
	Walking away from staff	2		12
Lindy	Staff friendly	3	5	60

Table 8.5. *Behaviour following speaking to a staff member*

Name	Behaviour following	Total	No. of observations of criterion	As %
Colin	Staff friendly	24	48	50
	Direct + indirect approaches to staff[a]	8		17
Carl	Staff friendly	47	89	53
	Speaking to staff	4		5
Alan	Staff friendly	21	39	54
	Speaking to staff	7		18
Keith	Staff friendly	26	60	43
	Speaking to staff	5		8
James	Staff friendly	44	87	51
	Speaking to staff	10		11
Nonny	Staff friendly	33	70	47
	Speaking to staff	8		11
Lindy	Staff friendly	29	51	57
	Speaking to staff	8		16

[a]Four of each.

kind of approach. Colin often had a staff friendly response but, as has already been seen, his approaches were quite often not successful, and, in such cases, he would try again. Keith, in contrast, would either try another approach or would speak to the staff member. Friendly responses from staff were not high in frequency. James would on occasion try a direct approach after an indirect one. As already established, he was almost assured of friendly attention following such an approach. Nonny showed a small number of avoidances of staff, walking away having first tried to approach a staff member. Lindy rarely attempted to approach staff indirectly, but generally received a friendly greeting when she did.

Behaviour following speaking to a staff member (Table 8.5). The children showed a comparatively uniform pattern of behaviour following speaking to a staff member. All the children most frequently had speech to staff followed by a staff friendly response. All but Colin would then go on to speak again. Colin, in contrast, would make some form of physical approach to the staff member. As he was the youngest child studied, and his language was not particularly well developed, he may have found this means of maintaining contact easiest. It is also possible, however, that since he was at times uncertain in his approaches, the act of speaking to the staff member 'broke the ice', so that he could go on to make an approach.

Behaviour directed towards other children

Behaviour following a head-turn towards another child (Table 8.6). It was not possible to include in the analysis all possible non-aggressive and aggressive outcomes of looks, approaches and speech to other children. For this reason, and due to the comparative rarity of aggressive behaviour, only non-aggressive outcomes have been included. For most of the children, looking at a child was followed by conversation with that child. Colin, however, again stands out as an exception, as Table 8.6 shows. He was most likely to look at a staff member, having looked at a child. Unlike the other children he would monitor the environment rather than going on to make contact. Both Alan and Keith showed a tendency to follow looking at a child with another head-turn towards a child.

Behaviour following an approach to another child (Table 8.7). The number of observations of approaches to other children were comparatively small. The most frequent subsequent behaviours for all the children were the other child speaking, speaking to the other child, and approaching the other child. It appears that examination of the behaviour following an approach to another child is not particularly fruitful.

Table 8.6. *Non-aggressive behaviour following a head-turn towards another child*

Name	Behaviour following	Total	No. of observations of criterion	As %
Colin	Head-turn towards staff	11	54	20
	Speaking to child	9		17
Carl	Speaking to child	7	31	23
	Approach to child	4		13
Alan	Speaking to child	5	17	29
	Head-turn towards child	2		12
Keith	Other child speaks	3	28	11
	Head-turn towards child	3		11
	Speaking to child	3		11
James	Other child speaks	2	19	11
	Approach to child	2		11
Nonny	Speaking to child	12	45	27
	Other child speaks	6		13
Lindy	Other child speaks	10	41	24
	Speaking to child	9		12

Table 8.7. *Non-aggressive behaviour following an approach to another child*

Name	Behaviour following	Total	No. of observations of criterion	As %
Colin	Other child speaks	3	17	18
	Head-turn towards child	3		18
	Speaking to child	3		18
Carl	Speaking to child	5	22	23
	Other child speaks	3		14
Alan	Approaching other child	1	8	13
	Speaking to child	1		13
Keith	Other child speaks	2	15	13
James	Speaking to child	8	16	50
Nonny	Speaking to child	9	33	27
	Other child speaks	8		24
Lindy	Other child speaks	1	7	14
	Approaching other child	1		14

Table 8.8. *Behaviour following speaking to another child*

Name	Behaviour following	Total	No. of observations of criterion	As %
Colin	Other child speaks	21	39	54
	Head-turn towards child	5		14
Carl	Other child speaks	20	44	45
	Speaking to child	9		20
Alan	Head-turn towards child	4	25	16
	Other child speaks	3		12
Keith	Direct approach to child	4	16	25
	Other child speaks	3		19
James	Speaking to child	8	43	19
	Other child speaks	6		14
Nonny	Other child speaks	43	116	37
	Speaking to child	20		17
Lindy	Other child speaks	23	70	33
	Speaking to child	15		21

Behaviour following speaking to another child (Table 8.8). The examination of the behaviour following this activity enables the child's effectiveness in eliciting interaction with other children to be seen. As the table shows, for Colin, more than half of the instances of his speaking to another child were followed by the other child speaking. Carl was also likely to be responded to in this way. Alan, however, most often followed speech to a child with a head-turn towards a child. Keith would most frequently speak to a child and then approach that child. James, Nonny and Lindy all showed a similar pattern: speech to a child would be followed either by further speech or by the speech of the other child. Differences can therefore be seen between the children in their ability to start and maintain a conversation with another child, and in the likelihood of them showing wary or watchful behaviours (head-turns) as did Colin and Alan.

Aggressive and antisocial behaviour. These forms of behaviour were so rarely seen that sequence analysis would not have yielded useful data. Incidents involving aggressive and antisocial acts appeared to be so infrequent that, for diagnostic purposes, it would probably be best for those using the technique diagnostically to keep a detailed account of such incidents, and to analyse cause and effect from this.

INTERCORRELATIONS OF APPROACH AND APPROACH-AVOIDANCE BEHAVIOUR

In addition to the analyses already outlined, a Pearson correlation matrix was calculated for all approaches and avoidance of others. Frequency data were used for this analysis. The aim of these correlations was to look for consistency in children's patterns of approaches to and approach-avoidance of staff and other children. One question of interest was whether those children who showed higher levels of ambivalence towards staff also showed higher levels of ambivalence in approaching children.

Approaches to and approach-avoidance of staff

A significant positive correlation was found between head-turns towards staff and head-turns away from staff ($r = -0.74$, $P = 0.03$). This would tend to indicate that children who were more watchful of staff were also more avoidant of them. There was a significant negative correlation between indirect approaches to staff and locomotor avoidance ($r = -0.77$, $P = 0.021$). A further negative correlation was found between locomotor avoidance of staff and backstepping approaches ($r = -0.75$, $P = 0.026$). It would appear, therefore, that the most indirect approaches to staff were negatively associated with locomotor avoidance. Hence the children who showed the more ambivalent approaches to staff tended not to be those who avoided them by walking away.

Approaches to and approach-avoidance of children

The frequency of head-turns towards other children was positively correlated with frequency of indirect approaches to them ($r = +0.92$, $P = 0.002$). This would tend to indicate a cautious strategy in approaching other children for some of the sample. In contrast, direct locomotor approaches to children were positively correlated with locomotor avoidance of them ($r = +0.77$, $P = 0.02$). These two findings taken together indicate that the children showed two possible strategies in making contact with one another: either watching and then sidling up, or approaching directly and then moving away again.

A comparison of the findings regarding staff and children

It had been suggested that patterns of approach to and approach-avoidance of staff might be repeated for approach to and approach-avoidance of other children. This did not appear to be the case. The children treated the staff and the other children very differently. A positive correlation of approach-avoidance of staff and direct approaches to children ($r = +0.68$, $P = 0.046$) indicated that for some of the sample ambivalence in approaching staff coexisted with considerable confidence in approaching other children. Approach-avoidance of other children was positively correlated with indirect approaches to staff ($r = +0.78$, $P = 0.018$) but was negatively correlated with locomotion away from staff ($r = -0.69$, $P = 0.04$). Overall there appeared to be little association between style of approach to staff and style of approach to children.

SUMMARY

The percentage and sequential data used in conjunction with each other allowed a fairly detailed picture to be drawn of the characteristics of individual children. Colin, Carl and Keith, for example, emerged as particularly watchful individuals. Lindy and Nonny were notable for the complementarity of their styles of interaction; James and Alan for their hostile behaviour. These were, perhaps, the most obvious findings. But closer examination of the observational data yielded more subtle findings: that, for example, Lindy was alone in not being approached and cuddled by a staff member, or that Alan's head-turns towards staff tended to go unnoticed and that he would then sidle up to staff members, a sequence of behaviour not seen in other children and one indicating a high degree of wariness of adults.

In a separate questionnaire study of the children, the Nursery Officers were asked about the children's characteristics, including watchfulness. Keith was not thought to be watchful, yet the observational data show that he spent a great deal of his time engaged in watchful behaviours. Observation thus provides a useful supplement to information which is already known about each child, particularly in the realm of ambivalent behaviours such as indirect approaches or approach-avoidance.

An important concern in the study of the development of abused children is the degree of aggression that they show. In the study reported in this chapter it was found that hostile behaviour was comparatively rare, as it was for most of the children described in Chapter 7. It is suggested that, where this kind of behaviour is of particular concern, it would be worth while making detailed observations of specific events in order to see how a child controlled – or failed to control – him- or herself in a tense and frustrating situation.

In order to be of use to the child care practitioner, observations such as the ones discussed above need to be seen in relation to all that is already known about the child and his or her background. Keith's markedly watchful behaviour, for example, may well be explicable in terms of the pleasure that his mother appeared to take in deliberately frightening him. These kinds of possibilities are discussed in the next chapter. Observation can be of particular value in highlighting behaviours that might well have gone unnoticed otherwise, as in Keith's case. Observation can also be useful in assessing the extent of a specific behaviour problem, as in James's case, and the efficacy of the forms of prevention used by staff.

9   Family life: bedtime and sexuality

In this chapter and the next we consider some of the material derived from the maternal interviews. The interview schedule, discussed in Chapter 4, is reproduced in the Appendix. The interviews were useful sources of information, but that information needs to be treated with caution. In any sample there are likely to be discrepancies between what mothers say they do as distinct from what they actually do; with this sample it is a particular difficulty. However, the interviews were useful to the extent that a mother talked about her child in a personal way and showed an awareness of that child's individuality and of his or her needs and feelings as distinct from her own. The interviews give us a picture of the child's life at home as well as areas of particular concern to the mother.

The information drawn from the interviews will be considered under five main headings here and in Chapter 10. In this chapter we look at two special issues which produced a wide range of responses from the mothers. First we examine the mothers' descriptions of a typical bedtime for the child, in which the mothers revealed a great deal about the quality of family life for their children. Secondly we look at the mothers' attitudes to the kinds of sex play that young children often take part in, and their reactions to questions about sexually related issues raised by their children. Considerable differences were found between the mothers, and there were hints of sexual misuse of two children in the responses to these questions.

In Chapter 10 we discuss firstly the extent to which the mothers appeared to enjoy their children as people, secondly the way in which affection was shown between mother and child, and thirdly the strategies that the mothers used in controlling their children, and their attitudes to different forms of punishment.

BEDTIME

The description of a typical bedtime for the child produced useful information on the mother's style of parenting. The information that a mother included – or, in some cases, omitted – gave some insight into the home life of the child. These questions were ones where the child, rather than the mother, was the focus of attention, and it is therefore possible that the responses were less skewed in the direction of social desirability.

The questions on bedtime run from number 62 to number 82 on the interview schedule (see Appendix) and cover bedtime routine in some detail. As before, responses to these questions are presented for each child in turn. In addition, the mother's reactions to bed-wetting (question 84) are included.

The descriptions of bedtimes have been grouped together under three headings:

1   'Special' bedtimes, where mothers mentioned some special bedtime routine (warmth, kiss and cuddle) that indicated an attempt to make bedtime special for the child.

2   'Difficult' bedtimes, where bedtimes were a source of conflict between parent and child, or parent and parent, or aggravated by poor housing conditions.

3   'Minimal caretaking' bedtimes, where bedtimes involved only the most basic caretaking on the part of the mother and appeared a cold, sad experience for the child.

'Special' bedtimes

Liz and Lindy
Lindy's bedtime was 7.30 p.m. This was generally adhered to whenever possible, but exceptions could be made for special events, and there was some flexibility. Lindy slept alone in her own room. Liz's description indicated that she generally tried to make bedtime fun for Lindy, that she usually read her a story, and that they always had a kiss and cuddle before Lindy went to sleep. No one else ever helped to put Lindy to bed. Lindy had a toy that the staff of the Family Centre had given her that she always took to bed. Liz thought that Lindy would make a considerable fuss if the toy could not be found one night. Once in bed, after her story and cuddle, the light would be put out, and Lindy was not allowed to get up and play in the bedroom. She had a nightlight, so that she did not sleep in complete darkness. She was given no food, drinks or sweets in bed.

If Lindy got up again she would be sent back to bed after a cuddle, when she would settle well. Lindy usually slept through the night, not needing to be lifted for a potty. On the occasions when Lindy woke in the night she would come quietly into her mother's bed, where she was allowed to stay. Although Liz had said, on a previous question, that Lindy slept through the night, on this question she commented that Lindy came into her bed every night. Late in the evening, if Lindy was awake and hungry, Liz would give her some food. Lindy had been out of nappies for a week, had wet the bed, and was now back in nappies again.

Jenny and James

James and his family had recently moved out of a room in a hotel they had lived in into a maisonette, where James had the luxury of his own bedroom. His regular bedtime was between 7.00 and 7.30 p.m. He could stay up a little later for special occasions, but then, or at weekends, he was usually in bed by 8.00 p.m. The bedtime routine was as follows:

'He just gets undressed, gets washed, puts his pyjamas on, says goodnight to us all and I take him up, tuck him in.'

Jenny's cohabitee would sometimes help to get James ready for bed, but James usually got himself ready. Affection was part of the routine, however, unlike the situation in many of the families studied:

James likes me to take him to bed, so he can give me a love and that. I have to lie down with him for about three seconds . . . I have to lie down with him, just put my head on his face. It's only for a few seconds, then he'll give me a tight hug and when I go he'll say 'You had a lie down a-a-all the time, didn't you?' He still says it and I've got to say it with him but he'll carry on going 'a-a-all' until I get out the door then he'll say 'All the time' . . . Some kids like bedtime stories, he likes to say that.

It could be argued that this kind of comment shows a much closer degree of meshing between parent and child than that seen in most other examples; a willingness on the mother's behalf to play along with her child's wishes, rather than simply expecting his conformity to hers.

James had a favourite pink teddy that he liked to take to bed; it had been his mother's. Jenny thought that he valued it particularly because of that. Once in bed, James was not allowed back up again. If he came out of his bedroom he was shouted at. He was allowed to have the light on and play with toys so long as he did not make a noise and wake the baby. He was not allowed food in bed, as he had been in the habit of hoarding biscuits behind the bed. He was not allowed sweets in bed now, although Jenny had used sweets as a bribe to make him stay in bed previously.

James would not cry if he woke in the night; he usually came into his mother's bed, as her cohabitee was working night-shifts. One night recently he had fallen out of his bed, so Jenny had taken him to hers. He had had nightmares when in the hotel, and his mother would try and comfort him:

Reassure him, you know, everyting's all right and that.

In response to the standard question on what the mother would do if her child got up in the night feeling chatty, Jenny gave a lively response:

Strangle him! No, get him to sleep. I'm nowty, me, when I have to wake up in the night unless it's for a reason, like he's upset. If I put him in my bed, he just goes to sleep.

James was allowed to sleep in his mother's bed all night if he wanted to. If he was hungry, Jenny wouldn't go downstairs to get him something to eat as she was too afraid of the dark. James occasionally wet the bed, but Jenny would not shout at him for this:

I don't shout at him because he'll do it in his sleep; it's only an accident.

Jenny felt that punishment would just make things worse.

'Difficult' bedtimes

Natalie and Nonny

Bedtime for Nonny appeared very different, and the effect of living in a single room with her mother was very clear. The previous night she had gone to bed between 8.00 and 8.30 p.m., but bedtime was frequently 10 or 11 o'clock, because of the housing arrangements. Natalie described bedtime in their previous house proudly, however.

When we used to be living in the house, she was in bed at half past seven. She used to take herself off to bed, honest to God. She was two and half years old, no, not even that, she was two, just left two, and she used to say 'Oh I'm tired.' She used to get the hot-water bottle what I had ready made her, she used to pick up her slippers and she used to go upstairs, and honest to God, she was fast asleep in her bed. And I used to leave the potty, it was full, she used to wee, so she had been up. And she was in bed and I used to go up and check her about an hour later. If ever she was crying, I used to go and check her.

Whilst Natalie clearly valued her daughter's independence, Nonny's bedtimes seemed a lonely time for the child. Now, in the flat, Natalie was forced into contact with the child at bedtime. She found the living arrangements a problem, as Nonny would watch television until very late, and it would frighten her, and she would sometimes wet the bed after watching a frightening programme. In the flat she had to share a bed with her mother; she had loved having a bed of her own. When asked whether her bed was a double one, Natalie replied:

No, it's a single board on the floor, like a divan board, with two back cushions from a settee . . . It's made into like a double bed if you put a single sheet, you know, a fitted sheet, and that makes it into a double bed, you know. It's on the floor though. We've got a single bed in the room but it's no use for the two of us . . . I sleep with her because, with it being a big bed, you know, and if the kiddie wakes up if she's frightened with it being a big bed. Well she's not frightened, but she likes to crawl near me . . . It's easy when she wets. I just wipe it underneath and the sheets dry dead quick. I mean, a lot of people put clean sheets on, but it's not worth it for just a little stain.

Natalie did not describe much of a bedtime routine. Nonny would wash herself, find her dummy, put her pyjamas on, give her mother a kiss and get into bed. She had no special toy that she took to bed. If she could not find her dummy, she could be comforted by her thumb instead. Once in bed, she

Table 9.1. *Mothers' attitudes to bedwetting*

Susan and Sally	No longer wets
Katherine and Kevin	Punitive. Took to doctor
Katherine and Keith	Verbally and physically chastised. Threatened with hospital
Elsie and Eddie	Mother angry. Verbally chastised
Winnie and William	Never wet. Bangs on door to be let out of bedroom at night
Connie and Carl	Unconcerned
Connie and Colin	Unconcerned
Andrea and Alan	Verbal chastisement. Threatened with nappies
Jenny and James	Unconcerned. Mother thinks punishment would only make matters worse
Natalie and Nonny	Unconcerned
Liz and Lindy	Put back in nappies. Unconcerned

would get out and play around the room again. She was not forced to stay in bed. If she made a noise and disturbed her mother's television viewing, however, she would be shouted at. If she woke up wanting a cuddle, Natalie would give her one. She would not give her food soon after bedtime, but late in the evening she would.

Nonny would often sleep through the night, but was sometimes given 'sleep medicine . . . because she is very active'. If she went to bed at around 9 o'clock she would usually sleep through: 'She's great like that.' Natalie would lift her for a potty most nights. She rarely woke or cried in the night. Natalie was not particularly concerned about bedwetting (Table 9.1).

Andrea and Alan

Andrea's account showed differences between her preferred bedtime routine with her children and that allowed by her husband. Alan had gone to bed at 6.30 p.m. the previous evening, because her husband had put him to bed. The following week, when her husband was at work, Andrea was going to let the children stay up until around 8 o'clock. At weekends they stayed up until 10.00 or 10.30 p.m. During the week, however, the children would not go to sleep as soon as they were put to bed:

Well, say they go to bed about half past six, it could still be 9 o'clock when I'm going up and down to stop them.

When at home, her husband liked them to have their tea and then go to bed, whereas Andrea preferred them to all be upstairs by 7.30 p.m. Alan shared a room with his brother, but had his own bed. Andrea's difficulty in getting them to bed came to the fore in her description of the bedtime routine:

They're moaning all the way upstairs, they don't want to go up to bed. Then I'll say, 'Come on, you've got to get in bed.' Then I'll put them in bed and they'll be running along the landing. Then I'll go up again, 'I want to go to the toilet', so I'm stood on the landing for about another half hour, let him go to the toilet. Then they'll get back in bed, then they'll get out a book – he'll always want to read.

Andrea's husband did not help in putting the children to bed. Alan had a teddy that he liked to take to bed when he was in the mood: 'It used to be Teddy and Snoopy the Dog at one time, but he lost that.' Andrea was one of the few mothers to mention one of her child's toys by name. She was also one of the few to spontaneously mention reading a story:

Well I give them a kiss every night, but if they ask for a cuddle, they sort of put their arms round me, and then they count themselves to ten and then I let them go . . . I don't know how they got into that habit, they just put their arms round me then count to ten then let me go, and sometimes I read them a story.

The children did not, however, necessarily settle down after this routine; they tended to jump around the room. They had once broken their bedroom lamp, so they only had light from the landing. Andrea felt that if they were allowed to play around, they would tire themselves out and sleep better. Andrea did not mind if they came back downstairs to her, if she was alone. They had to go back to bed before their father came home. If Alan was hungry he could come downstairs for food if Andrea was alone, but not if father was at home. Alan generally slept through the night, and was not allowed into his parents bed:

He used to come into our bedroom and with me being tired, the automatic thing was to open the covers, let him get in, snuggle him up and get him back to sleep again, but my husband likes him to go back into his own bed.

Sent back to his own room, Alan would cry and make a fuss. Andrea would go and see to him, whereas her husband would shout at him to shut up. For this reason, Andrea would sometimes get into Alan's bed with him. Andrea's account indicated her difficulty in keeping the children from annoying her husband. Whilst she appeared sensitive to the children, she did not exert a great deal of control over them at times, so that she needed to spend hours each evening putting them to bed. The children also experienced an inconsistent environment, depending upon whether their father was home or not. With regard to bedwetting, Andrea had told Alan that he was naughty, and also threatened to put him back into nappies, which upset him.

Susan and Sally
Susan usually got Sally ready for bed between 7.00 and 8.00 p.m. She had her nightdress warming on the radiator and if she was busy her husband would sometimes undress Sally for her. Sally then lay down on the couch and might not fall asleep until 9.30 or 10.00 p.m. Susan and her husband experienced considerable difficulty with Sally's bedtime:

The only thing is you can't get her to go to bed. She's got to fall asleep on the couch first and then you've got to carry her up. She goes in her own bed but you've got to carry her up there. She won't go to bed. She never has since she was a baby. We've just got her in her own bed now. And she's never wet the bed. She used to sleep in with me till she was about two. I tried her in her own bed but she'd go in her bed and she'd maybe be sleeping and then during the night she'd be in yours. She gets up and goes to the toilet on her own and everything, she always has, never wet the bed.

Control of the situation had effectively passed from the parent to the child and Susan felt powerless to change things. Sally had now, at 4, graduated to her own bed in her parents' room, but they could not persuade her to sleep in her own bedroom, which had been prepared for her for some time. If Sally woke in the evening she came back downstairs and her parents waited for her to fall asleep on the couch again before carrying her back up to bed.

Sally was allowed to have cereal and a drink if she wanted them but not sweets. Susan was prepared to be very flexible about letting her play with toys in bed or read, if only Sally would go to bed:

Oh aye she can play with them. If she'd go to bed I'd let her play with them – that's the only hard bit, if I could get her to go to bed.

Sally did not have any special routine although her mother mentioned that just recently she had been taking one of her dolls to bed with her. Susan was full of anecdotes about Sally:

Like this morning before we came out, she put it [the doll] in the bed and said to her 'I'm going to the nursery now, don't cry . . . I'll be back in a minute.'

If Sally woke in the night in distress, Susan said she just left her, but on further questioning it transpired that Sally got into her parents' bed and went to sleep. Susan did not mind that, but felt at a loss as to how to proceed further with instigating a bedtime routine:

I mean it'd be alright if we could only get her just to go to bed early.

'Minimal caretaking' bedtimes

Elsie and Eddie

Eddie always went to bed at 6 o'clock and was not allowed to stay up longer if he was not tired. He had his own room. No one else helped with his bedtime and Eddie seemed more or less to take himself off to bed. Elsie might help him to get undressed, then Eddie went to the toilet and then to bed. They did not have any special bedtime rituals but Elsie mentioned that Eddie always took a particular, favourite teddy to bed with him. She painted rather a sad picture of this little boy in bed:

He just gets hold of his teddy and clings in his arms with it.

Elsie made no mention of any bedtime kiss or cuddle, and in fact elsewhere in the interview complained of Eddie's clinging behaviour.

Eddie was not allowed to get up once he had gone to bed and he went to sleep with the light on, because he was frightened of the dark. He could have a drink if he was thirsty but Elsie did not like him having anything to eat, although she might let him have a slice of toast if he was really hungry. If Eddie woke crying, Elsie said she might sit him on her knee for a bit, but she did not allow him to get into her bed and she would not get into his.

Elsie lifted Eddie for a potty in the night and was upset if he wet the bed:

Well sometimes I get a bit mad about it you know, 'cos I have to keep changing him about four times a day . . . and that's a pile of washing for me.

Winnie and William
Winnie and William had no special bedtime ritual. William went to bed at 7 o'clock and Winnie was not prepared to be flexible about bedtime. She expected William to go to bed when he was told and by and large he did. Sometimes he undressed himself, sometimes Winnie helped, but no one else helped to get him ready. William took a book to bed with him and Winnie was not aware of any special toy that he might have. Sometimes Winnie might read him a story, 'but if he's naughty I don't bother'.

Winnie would leave a drink of orange by his bed but no food. She said she just ignored it if William got up once he was supposed to be in bed, but on further questioning it transpired that William could not get out of his room:

He can't 'cos the door's shut. Well not really, no, 'cos it's one of those twist-a-ball ones. He doesn't know how to turn it 'cos it's a bit stiff. I just shut it and he can't get out.

If William wanted to go to the toilet he banged on the door. Winnie lifted him for a potty during the night and claimed he never wet the bed: 'he's very clean'. She also said that William never woke up crying in the night and that he was never frightened. If he were to wake she would just ignore it. She certainly would not let him get in her bed ('he's too big') and she would not get in his, although she conceded that she might sit on his bed.

Connie and Carl (first interview)
Connie claimed she was very strict on bedtime and always had been. Carl went to bed at 7 o'clock and Connie was not prepared to be flexible about this unless they had all gone out somewhere and were back late. Carl shared a bedroom with his brother Colin. Connie undressed them in front of the television and then Carl

sort of drinks it [bottle], sits down for a bit and he'll say 'I'm going to bed now Mummy' and he's off. He's in bed and that's it – the works – I just go up to him, tuck him in and that's it.

There was no special bedtime ritual or toy. Carl was not allowed to play in bed, he did not get anything to eat or drink, and the light was switched off.

Connie said Carl did not get up in the night but that Colin did. It emerged whilst discussing bedtime that Carl frequently screamed at night and Connie seemed to accept this:

I just leave him. He's always done it. He's always done it you know. Colin's started it now. I don't bother.

At bedtime Connie sometimes sat with them and read to them, but this did not appear to be a pleasant experience for the boys:

. . . that's how I started them going to bed theirselves – by sitting in the room and reading a book, you know. Instead of shouting at them I'd just ignore them by reading [aloud]. They'd just drop off, they were that fed up.

Connie said that Carl sometimes wet the bed but that she was not particularly bothered about this as he had only been out of nappies for a couple of months.

Connie and Carl (second interview)

Bedtime was 7 o'clock. Carl would not allow his father to help to put him to bed; it had to be his mother. He often took toy cars to bed, but was not particularly attached to these. If he tried to get up in the night he was smacked. He generally cried upon waking in the night, and Connie would, she said, cuddle him. This seemed inconsistent, when considering her earlier response. She did not know why he cried. Carl occasionally wet the bed, but Connie was not particularly concerned by this.

Connie and Colin

Colin's bedtime was 6.30 p.m. with no flexibility allowed. He was, Connie said, always tired out by then.

I'd love them to be awake longer but by that time they're absolutely shattered, so what can I do?

Colin would have a bottle and then put himself to bed. No one else helped put him to bed. He had a favourite doll that he liked to take to bed. Other than his bottle, there appeared to be no other shared routine. Connie said that she read them a story at night. However, according to the previous interview, this was not a particularly jolly occasion; she would read until the children were so bored that they could stay awake no longer. The children had indirect light in their room, and would play until tired. Colin was occasionally allowed back into the room where his parents were. He rarely slept through the night, and would cry on waking. Connie would make him a drink. Again, Connie presented a picture of minimal caretaking at bedtime. With regard to bedwetting, Connie was just leaving it.

Katherine and Kevin

Kevin usually went to bed at 7.30 p.m., although Katherine did say that she let him stay up longer on Friday and Saturday nights. His brother Keith went much earlier as he was 'gone' by 7 o'clock. Kevin was sharing a double bed with his maternal uncle, who was staying with the family at the time. There were only two bedrooms and Keith and the baby were both in with Katherine and her husband. Katherine would have liked Kevin and Keith to share a bedroom.

The evening routine was bath when they got home, into pyjamas, something to eat, a play and then bed. If the weather was nice they might be allowed to play out in the small back garden before their bath. Katherine's husband was not allowed to help with the children. He was an epileptic and Katherine discouraged him from helping in case he had a fit whilst doing so.

There was no special bedtime routine or ritual for Kevin, although Katherine said she would 'just give him a kiss'. Kevin took a police car to bed with him:

He only has that little play and he's out in 5 minutes – it's just a comfort to him.

Kevin was not allowed to get up and play once he had gone to bed and was only allowed to play with toys in bed in the mornings if his parents were still in bed. He would go to bed with the light on and Katherine would turn it off when he was asleep. If Kevin woke in the night and was thirsty, Katherine would give him a drink but nothing to eat.

Katherine said that if Kevin woke in the night he just lay there and did not cry, but then went on to say that she would not know if he woke up frightened or was crying because they were in separate rooms so she would not notice. She did not appear to be particularly concerned about this. She was more concerned about the fact that Kevin had had a dummy at night until well past his fourth birthday and that she had great difficulty getting him to give it up; Also that he was bedwetting. It did not appear to have occurred to Katherine that there might be an emotional basis for both of these. She had taken Kevin to the doctor about his bedwetting as she thought there was something wrong with him, but said the doctor had told her that either Kevin was lazy or that he could not control himself. Katherine claimed Kevin had improved recently and thought this was because she had started training Keith and 'Keith was great . . . and he was getting all the praise'. (This optimism about Keith's toilet training was to be short lived, as can be seen in the following interview.)

Katherine and Keith

Keith generally went to bed at 6.30 p.m., with no flexibility, although he would be allowed to play in bed if not tired. Keith now shared a bed with his brother.

The extent of Katherine's bedtime caretaking was to wash the two boys, get them into their pyjamas and give them a drink, then make sure that they had been to the toilet. Her husband did not usually help. Keith had a teddy that he took to bed: 'He doesn't play with it, it's just at night-time.' Katherine also said that she would throw them on the bed, a routine activity, 'just one throw'. Once in bed they were not allowed to get out, but could play in bed.

If Keith got up, his treatment would depend on the reason. If he was frightened, he would be allowed to stay up for a while. If just feeling chatty, he would be sent back to bed. If Keith woke in the night, he would usually cry.

He'd probably get up and come into our room if he's got the courage to walk through the dark. I think he'd cry.

Katherine thought that he did not often wake up. He was sometimes frightened by monsters in the dark – the only child whose mother had reported such fears:

Like if I had something on the wardrobe, hanging on the wardrobe, a shadow on the wall. It was a monster to him, that . . . I've got to make sure there's nothing, no shadow or anything on the wall.

Bedwetting was a serious problem for Katherine at that time; Keith was wetting the bed nightly, far more frequently than other mothers had reported.

I've smacked him for it but its's a waste of time . . . sometimes I wake and think shall I get up and get him out for a wee, but I'm too tired, I can't get out of bed. But I used to do that with him . . . I've told him off, I've told him I'll take him to the hospital. I've frightened him once. It's a waste of time, he still does it so.

Katherine would not be drawn on the way that she had frightened him. She attributed the bedwetting to cold weather, and to the fact that little boys 'wee nearly every hour, every half hour or two hours'. From this part of the interview it appeared that Keith was quite frightened at bedtime, and it is also possible that his bedwetting was attributable to his fear of walking about the house in the dark, so that he could not go to the toilet. Katherine did not appear to have made any major concessions to his fear of the dark. He was allowed into bed with his parents, but appeared to be too frightened to get there.

COMMENTS

Where the children had 'special' bedtimes, the mother's skills in warm parenting became most evident. The stories, special cuddles and routines showed a degree of warmth that was often reflected in comments about other times of the day. More common, however, were difficult bedtimes, or bedtimes which involved minimal caretaking.

With the exception of Natalie and Nonny, for whom one-room living appeared to be the main problem, a lack of consistency and absence of clear guidelines appeared to be the chief sources of difficulty. For Andrea and Alan, the bedtime routine was determined by whether or not Alan's father was at home, and bedtime ranged from 6.30 to 10.30 p.m. Sally, too, would be ready for bed by 7 o'clock, but then controlled the time that she went to bed. Carl and Colin were largely ignored at bedtime; even their bedtime story was a way of ignoring them for Connie. Bedtime was bleak for William, shut in his room to keep him out of harm's way, and bleak also for Keith, fearful of monsters and too afraid to make his way through the dark to his parents' room.

The attitudes that the mothers expressed in talking about bedtime seemed to capture the essence of much of what they said about their children at other times of the day. It was our feeling that asking about times such as this, where there were no obvious expectations on our part, formed a particularly valuable part of the interview.

SEXUALLY RELATED ISSUES

In the course of the interview the mothers were asked how they felt about their child playing with his or her genital area, and about tolerance of children's sexually related play. They were also asked whether the child saw either parent naked and about basic sexual information that the child might have. It was anticipated that the parents would vary considerably in their attitudes concerning this rather sensitive area, and this indeed proved to be the case. It was also felt that responses to these questions reflected aspects of the mothers' attitudes to their children. Some mothers were relatively tolerant and easy-going, whilst others were more anxious or punitive. A small number of mothers described their children in ways that provoked some concern on our behalf, although no mother described sexual abuse of a child *per se*.

The mothers's attitudes are summarised in Tables 9.2 to 9.5. The majority of the mothers said little on the subject, answering in a matter-of-fact way as they had done on other aspects of the child's daily routine. Andrea said, for example, when asked whether Alan played with himself, that she did not know if he did, and that if he did, she was unsure how she would feel:

I don't know. The Welfare, they always said it was natural you know, so I've had talks like that and they've said you shouldn't sort of keep telling them off because when they get older they'll think 'Oh well, I shouldn't be doing that.'

Several of the mothers had consulted professionals, and Andrea's comments were typical of the responses of many of the mothers. Some had already resolved this issue for themselves in relation to older siblings.

In general, the mothers tended to be unconcerned about self-exploration, or about their child seeing other children undressed. In general, too, they tended to try to ignore their children if they giggled about such things. Most of the

Table 9.2. *Mothers' attitudes to genital exploration*

Susan and Sally	Not bothered
Katherine and Kevin	Said he used to do it but does not now. Not bothered
Katherine and Keith	Does not like it, told him to stop. Went and watched through crack in doorway
Elsie and Eddie	He does not do it, and mother would not like it if he did
Winnie and William	Does not like it. Would try and keep him covered up
Connie and Carl	Does not mind. Tells him it is naughty but would not punish. Claimed he circumcised himself as a baby and made himself sore and septic
Connie and Colin	Does not mind
Andrea and Alan	Unsure. Welfare said to leave it, in relation to Alan's older brother
Jenny and James	Would not do anything. Leaving it
Natalie and Nonny	Does not mind: 'she's just experiencing and has to know what it's like'

Table 9.3. *Mothers' attitudes to children going to the toilet together, giggling about the toilet and seeing other children undressed*

Susan and Sally	Takes no notice: 'She's not too bad'
Katherine and Kevin	Ignores if giggling about toilet: 'We find it a bit funny, me and our kid [Katherine's brother].' Does not allow to go to toilet together. Does not mind siblings and friends being undressed together
Katherine and Keith	As above
Elsie and Eddie	Would not mind
Winnie and William	Does not like them to go to toilet together, but does not mind if siblings and friends undressed together
Connie and Carl	Mother finds it funny
Connie and Colin	Takes no notice
Andrea and Alan	Alan finds it funny to 'pooh sitting down and wee standing up'; mother not bothered. Baths with sister
Jenny and James	In hostel: 'the children there were dirty . . . just filthy messing about in the toilet'. Embarrassed at children undressed together
Natalie and Nonny	Takes no notice: 'If they find it funny, let them find it funny'

mothers were less keen on children going to the toilet together, and would not allow this. There was considerable variation between the families in relation to seeing their parents undressed. Most of the mothers were relaxed about this, and several would bath with their children. Winnie and Elsie did not like their sons to see them undressed. Both Katherine and Connie had changed their attitudes in the course of the year between interviews, Katherine not allowing Keith to see her undressed, although Kevin had done so, and Connie feeling less happy about her sons seeing her undressed than she had done previously.

Table 9.4. *Mothers' attitudes to child seeing parents undressed*

Susan and Sally	Baths with either parent
Katherine and Kevin	Sees parents undressed
Katherine and Keith	Has not seen either parent undressed. Mother bothered about this
Elsie and Eddie	Does not see mother undressed
Winnie and William	'I don't dress in front of him – well, he's a lad – he's not a baby any more'
Connie and Carl	Baths with mother
Connie and Colin	Sees both parents undressed. This bothers mother
Andrea and Alan	Baths with either parent
Jenny and James	Sees both parents undressed. Does not mind
Natalie and Nonny	Sees mother undressed, also father when at home. Used to bother mother. Nonny says 'Oh cover up your milk bottles'

Table 9.5. *Child's knowledge of reproduction, if any*

Susan and Sally	'She'll maybe know – she knows everything else'
Katherine and Kevin	Told when pregnant. He thought it funny
Katherine and Keith	Would tell, but has not asked. Did not believe mother was carrying baby when explained
Elsie and Eddie	'No, he's too young. I'd just say they come out of my belly'
Winnie and William	Told when pregnant: 'He could see it'
Connie and Carl	'Yes, he's well advanced. I'll be a granny before he's 16'
Connie and Colin	Learned from TV
Andrea and Alan	6-year-old sister explained 'in a nice way'
Jenny and James	Mother explained when pregnant
Natalie and Nonny	Learned with mother from book

In the following sections we present quotations of particular interest, drawn from interviews where mothers talked at length about these issues. The quotations deal, in the main, specifically with the issue of genital self-exploration, as this produced some noteworthy comments. Most of the mothers expressed little in the way of opinions on the subject; all replies are summarised in the tables. In considering the comments quoted here, it is worth bearing in mind that Nonny, Kevin and Keith were the children who were most likely to have experienced sexual misuse. Natalie had been asked by a boyfriend to make Nonny watch them have sex, and since Natalie and Nonny lived in one room together and Natalie was sexually very active, Nonny was quite likely to have seen at least some sexual activity. Kevin shared a bed with his uncle (his mother's brother), and there were some some suspicions of an incestous relationship between his mother and uncle. Natalie and Katherine were the two mothers who talked most freely about their children's self-exploration. Two other mothers, Jenny and Susan, gave responses to the questions that afforded insight into their high degree of sensitivity to their children's development.

Natalie and Nonny
Natalie said that she would not mind if Nonny played with herself:

... she's experiencing. She's got to know what it's like. She doesn't know where things are or anything like that. She does sometimes lift up her top and she'll say 'Oh I've got boobs like mummy, but I don't need a bra yet', but she never does touch herself. I mean, if she does, I mean, they've got to know they are. I mean, she has asked me once or twice what it is you know, but I just say to her, you know, give her little things, you know ... I'm very shy. Well if she messes about down there, I say 'That's your pussy', but I shouldn't have said that because she tells [another mother] 'Mummy's got a pussy like your pussy' – she's talking about the cat. My mum said to say 'money box' and I said no chance because she'll put money in it, so I had to start thinking, what the hell, she did, she put money in it once ... my mum gave her some money once and she said 'Oh I'll put it in the money box.' It was very embarrassing when she lifted up her skirt. She stood there, pulled down her bloody knickers. I just burst out laughing ... she knows, she always calls them boobs, either boobs or milk bottles – especially milk bottles. She says 'Oh I'm going to have milk bottles like mum's when I'm older.' I thought I haven't got big ones, but she always says big ones. She gets my bras and tries them on as well. Stuffs them with socks.

Katherine and Kevin
Katherine talked about Kevin going to the toilet with other children in reply to a different question: 'Is there any sort of play you don't allow?'

The only thing I don't let them do is go to the toilet together or things like that. He'll say 'Come on Keith' and I say 'Where are you going' and he says 'I'm going to the toilet' and I say 'No you're not, you go on your own', you know. I mean you can't do it when you're older so you may as well stop it now.

Kevin used to play with himself, but did not now. When asked whether there was anything else that he did as a habit when overtired or worried, she replied:

The only thing he does – he done the other night was – we got him up, for a wee and he was still asleep and he was like this [demonstrated whole hand movement bringing fingers together in a plucking action]. I don't know what he was doing, picking things off the bed you know. We was laughing, you know, me and our kid [Katherine's brother], 'cos what did he do – he sat up – 'cos he was still sat up in bed and he was like this. But he's terrible when we wake him up, he doesn't know what he's doing. You've got to guide him to the potty, hold the potty, hold the potty and hold his, you know, thingy to do it, 'cos he's, you know – you can't wake him up.

It seems that despite her beliefs stated earlier, Katherine and her brother had both appeared to derive a certain degree of voyeuristic pleasure from Kevin's nocturnal behaviour. The extent of this was not clear, but her comments about Keith quoted below indicated that her sons' sexuality was a continuing source of fascination to her. Asked about children playing together when undressed she said that she and 'our kid' found it funny when her sons played with her niece in this way, but

we don't let them carry on and all you know. But me dad gets mad – so he says to me one day, 'You're going to get into trouble one day you are if he does it outside.'

Again, her meaning is not altogether clear.

Katherine and Keith
Katherine had noticed that Keith played with himself, and did not like it:

I don't like it. It's the way he does it you know. I was like cleaning up at the weekend . . . I thought 'Where has he gone?', and I looked, and I think it was shock more than anything and I said 'What are you doing down there?' He went dead red you know. He said nothing and started crying. I walked away and went out down the hall and had a look through the crack and he was there, looking. Kevin used to do it a lot but I didn't think he would pick it up because Kevin was doing it while he was younger . . . it kind of shocked me and I was dead embarrassed.

When asked whether she had told Keith off about it, Katherine answered:

I just said 'Leave it alone, that's enough now.' He said 'I'm not doing anything mum.' Well it was all stuck up and everything. Have you ever seen it, have you ever seen little boys like that?

Katherine's return to look at Keith through the crack in the door, and her invitation to the interviewer to enter into conversation on the subject demonstrated a degree of interest not shown by the other mothers, and added to the feelings of discomfort that we had about the issue of sexuality in relation to this family.

Jenny and James
James did not play with himself, as far as Jenny was aware. If he did so, she said she wouldn't do anything, but mentioned an incident some time previously when she found James engaged in sexual play with a little girl. In describing this episode, and also James's learning about reproduction, she showed a sensitivity to her child unusual for this group of mothers:

I used to be embarrassed, 'cos I've seen him messing about with this little girl. I was embarrassed about it – I thought my son, do that. He was only exploring. I would stop him from doing it in case he hurt himself, but I wouldn't let him think it was rude because it's not.

When asked whether James knew where babies come from yet, Jenny answered:

Oh yes. When I was pregnant with the baby, I got twenty questions. And now, like when I came out of hospital with baby and I was losing it for so long, well he saw it once. He came in the bathroom and I was changing you see, and every time I go to the toilet he'll say 'You're not bleeding today mum' – you know, things like that. But I don't bother because I know sooner or later it's going to be explained to him. I'm trying now to explain, so that when he's older I don't have to go right through it all . . . he knows everything, even how babies get there. I was very embarrassed when he shouted it out on a bus when I was pregnant . . . he said 'I know where they come from but how did the baby get there?' I was so embarrassed and said 'Get over here' and everyone was looking at me and laughing . . . I just said 'Ask your dad', but I told him myself and he just thought it was rather funny.

Susan and Sally
Sally was interested in 'titties'.

She's going through the stage right now. What was it, last night, she says 'I've got titties' and I says 'Oh?' And if you see it on the television, sometimes you'll say 'Look at that woman, she's got a big bust', and Sally'll say to you 'That's naughty big bust.'

When asked whether Sally ever saw either of her parents undressed, Susan replied:

Yeah she goes in the bath with me. She goes in the bath with her dad. She's done it since she was a baby anyway. She washes your back. I mean the only job is trying to get her hair washed. She's not bad, she likes the water – it's just her hair. Last night I let her wash her own hair – well I let her wet it – so she comes downstairs and says to her dad 'I've washed my hair.' I let her wet it herself so she wet it all. So she never cried last night 'cos I let her wet her own hair. I've got her started now using the hairdrier. She used to be scared of the hairdrier – you know on her head. Now I've got her – I can use it on her now. 'Cos I used to show her doing it on mine first. Then I says to her, 'It don't burn you know.' I says to her, 'Feel it against your hand, it don't burn you.' So now she'll sit and let you do it with her hair.

These comments on Sally's hairwashing and drying showed a gentleness and patience not generally apparent in the comments made by the mothers. It is likely that Susan developed the idea of letting Sally wet her own hair from suggestions made at the Family Centre, and she had clearly built these kinds of ideas into her behaviour with her child.

COMMENTS

Again, this section shows the information that can be derived from asking a series of comparatively innocuous questions about an issue which all parents of young children have to confront. Whilst it can be difficult to address the question of sexual abuse directly in intervention with a family, the responses given to these questions opened up this area comparatively easily. Particularly noteworthy was Katherine, who appeared to talk freely about her sons in a way which might raise concern over potential sexual misuse of the children. A comment like Connie's that Carl had circumcised himself as a baby and made himself sore, also merits closer attention.

As with the accounts of bedtime and comments on bedwetting, the mothers' responses showed up some rather different attitudes to their children, and to what is a normal activity for a young child. Some mothers were generally unconcerned and saw them as normal parts of growing up, others were concerned about specific issues, whilst yet others were more clearly punitive. It is possible that some mothers in this position could benefit from access to more information on normal aspects of child development, perhaps in some kind of structured format.

10 Affection and control

In this chapter we examine some of the information gleaned from the maternal interviews around the areas of affection, discipline and control. As we have seen in Chapter 9, the interviews provide a picture of what the child's life at home was like as well as highlighting areas of particular concern to the mothers. Many mothers appeared unaware of the effect of their own behaviour on their child even in everyday situations. They often failed to take the child's feelings and intentions into account. They were particularly worried about controlling and disciplining their children and tended to favour physical punishment rather than what we characterise below as a more low-profile approach of using concessions and bargaining with the child. All the mothers said they smacked their children but none of them believed that smacking children did them any good. Some said they found it difficult to control themselves when they used physical punishment. Mothers tended to be inconsistent, which must be confusing for a child, and many admitted using emotional punishment, threatening that they would stop loving the child, or would send the child away.

The mothers' replies to questions are considered here in terms of:

1. Enjoyment of the child as a person/appreciation of the child's personality and individuality.
2. Affection
3. Strategies of punishment and control

ENJOYMENT OF THE CHILD AS A PERSON/APPRECIATION OF THE CHILD'S PERSONALITY AND INDIVIDUALITY

As a preamble to the questions on discipline and control (see Appendix) the mothers were asked two questions on positive aspects of their relationships with their children. The first of these was: 'I wonder if you could tell me how you and [child's name] get on with each other? What sorts of things do you particularly enjoy in him/her?' Such a question gives a mother a chance to talk about what her child is actually like rather than simply focussing on what he or she can and cannot do, should and should not do. It can also give an indication of the quality of the mother–child relationship: the sorts of things they enjoy

150

doing together, the shared pleasures that compensate for the daily grind of caring for a pre-schooler. This question was also trying to probe whether the mothers had an awareness of their own child's individuality. It is important for a child's development that parents see their child as a distinct and likeable personality, an individual with his or her own likes and dislikes, age-related needs, and feelings. When this does not happen, and the child is seen primarily as being there to fulfill the parents' needs or as a reflection of the parents' own, often low, self-esteem, the child's needs and rights are neglected and his or her development suffers as a consequence. A dramatic example of this was afforded in the previous chapter when Natalie described how her boyfriend wanted 3-year-old Nonny to witness their sexual intercourse.

Most parents can provide countless anecdotes about their children. It is interesting to note that many of these mothers were unable to think of positive, particular examples of what they enjoyed in their children. Their replies are presented under four headings: (1) positive, personal; (2) impersonal; (3) reflection on negative attributes; (4) inappropriate, or unable to give examples.

1. Positive, personal

Susan and Sally

Susan was one of the few mothers spontaneously to recount many anecdotes about her child throughout the interview, and it was possible to recognise the lively, bright child, who dominated the playroom when in attendance, in her mother's stories of what she did at home, her funny sayings, her play etc. Susan particularly enjoyed Sally's sense of humour:

When she has a laugh. Sometimes she'll come in, you know, and she'll say some comical things to you . . . Oh she pretends she's got a dog sometimes. She'll say 'Come on' to the dog. That was through me. One day I was having a laugh with her and I said to her 'Come on, poor dog. It's a shame, it's got a lost home, Sally.' Now she does it.

Liz and Lindy

Liz listed several things that she enjoyed in her child. In particular, she liked her company, and going on trips to the park with her.

Andrea and Alan

Andrea was one of the mothers who emphasised facial attributes:

It's the expression on his face you know. I feel like sometimes I could just pick him up and cuddle him. I don't know, he just does something to me.

Unlike the remarks of some other mothers, however, this comment did not have a sting in the tail; there was no mention of negative attributes, and no reflection of disliked behaviour.

Jenny and James
Jenny found many things to comment on in her child, all of them positively valued by her. She gave perhaps the most unusual set of examples, which appear to indicate considerable enjoyment of her child as a person.

His imagination – and I can talk to him now, I can have a conversation you know, a proper conversation with him. Like we've got this mortgage, and we came in here last week and he told the staff 'We've got a mortgage, we're moving' . . . You know, I think he's got to the stage where I think he's dead funny – even if he's done things that you think are bad. Like when I took him to the park yesterday, he was holding Carol's hand and he walked past these two fellows on the grass and he shouted 'You've got big titties Carol.'

2. Impersonal

Katherine and Kevin
Katherine talked of there being a special bond between herself and Kevin but nowhere did she talk about his individual qualities or give any picture of what her child was really like as a person.

You see there's been a difference with me and him – we're close – he was me first baby and everything. I mean he was. I don't know, there is a bond there. I just can't explain it, but he gets a lot, a lot more than Keith does as, you know, regards sweets and things like that. Not in front of Keith 'cos Keith is already in bed like, but he tends to get more bought for him. No offence to Keith, I mean Keith gets everything he wants, but when he's not there he [Kevin] seems to, you know, to be there when you're getting something like or, you know, having something.

3. Reflection on negative attributes

Katherine and Keith
Katherine gave a brief mention of two things that she liked about Keith before going on to comment on negative attributes, then her own preoccupations.

The way he talks, the way he sings and dances, things like that. He's been a bit difficult. When he was born, like, he was premature and they took him off me and put him in the In-Care Unit like . . . It was about four days before I even held him proper. I think there was something missing there you know. Then he went into care so I didn't have much to do with him. I've not really had much to do with him really, then he's been in here.

Natalie and Nonny
Natalie valued her child's looks – she was indeed a particularly pretty little girl – but she qualified her comments. Even in a description of Nonny's good points, Natalie reflected on negative aspects of behaviour:

I don't know really . . . I mean, I like her when she's sitting there smiling and that. I mean, she's got a beautiful smile. I mean, she pulls a little face when she laughs and that . . . She makes me laugh – when she's not naughty.

4. Inappropriate, or unable to give examples

Elsie and Eddie
When asked what she particularly liked about Eddie, Elsie complained about him being a 'clinger'. Eddie, a bright child with a lively comic talent, was a favourite in the Family Centre, but his mother could have been talking about a different child and she painted a bleak picture of their life together:

Well he's a clinger. He clings. He wants loving all the time and he'll come up to me and say 'I want a love'. You see when I've smacked him – and I smack him and smack him and smack him again and I can't control it sometimes, you know with this thing going on. That's why I've come here today to see A. [her social worker]. I mean this morning I smacked him really hard and I didn't mean to – just did it. But sometimes we do fight. But he's sometimes he's a bit out of hand, he's demanding all the time.

Winnie and William
Winnie, when asked what she particularly enjoyed in William, replied 'everything'. She was unable to give any more specific examples and there were no anecdotes and few descriptions of William's individual qualities in any of her other replies. When asked how they got on together she said:

All right. He's happy.

Connie and Carl (first interview)
Connie could not really think of what she particularly liked about Carl, and all she would say was that she liked reading to him.

Connie and Colin
Connie also had difficulty in thinking of anything that she liked about her other son:

I don't know. I've no idea . . . That I don't like, his whingeing. That I do like? His obedience.

Again, this mother laid emphasis on negative qualities, having had a hard time thinking of any positive attributes. The only attribute mentioned, obedience, although highly adaptive on the child's behalf, would not be expected to be the major positive attribute of a 3-year-old.

Connie and Carl (second interview)
When asked for her opinions concerning aspects of Carl that she enjoyed, Connie's only comment was 'Everything', which was fairly uninformative and might be taken as indicating the opposite.

AFFECTION

The second question on more positive aspects of the mother–child relationship asked how freely parent and child showed affection to one another. This question could have been more likely to produce biased answers as the mothers would have some expectation that the interviewer might have clear views on this topic. The mothers' replies are grouped under two headings: (1) parent and child showed affection freely to each other/mother describes herself as warm towards her child; (2) parent and child did not show affection freely to each other.

1. Parent and child showed affection freely/mother warm

Susan and Sally
Susan replied:

Yeah, we're not too bad really. It's just when she goes in one of her moods 'cos she can't get her own way see, she takes it out on me ... Yeah we muck about a lot. Like she had chewing gum yesterday and I had chewing gum and she says 'Blow a bubble' and she's banging it on my face!

Liz and Lindy
Liz described herself as 'warm' towards Lindy, but said no more.

Natalie and Nonny
Natalie said that she and Nonny kissed and cuddled a lot.

Andrea and Alan
With Alan, Andrea said that a routine had been developed:

When he comes home at night from the Nursery and I come and sit down, his first thing is automatic straight at the side of me.

Jenny and James
Jenny simply answered 'Yes' to the question, but went on to say in response to the following one, 'I think that especially when there's another baby on the scene you need to', showing a sensitivity to James's needs. She went on to comment on the lack of affection in her own childhood, and that of her cohabitee, saying that she wanted to give James a different experience.

2. Parent and child did not show affection freely

Winnie and William
Winnie's reply indicated that William would have liked more affection from her than she was prepared to give:

No. Sometimes he gets a bit soppy but I say 'You're too big for that now – you're a big boy. Big boys don't do that.' He's too old. He's getting a bit too old for it now. He's getting too . . . they go soft when you do that.

Connie and Carl
Connie said she tried to show affection to Carl but that he was not interested: 'I try, but I think he's very reserved at the moment. Elsewhere in the interview she commented:

He's going through a stage of wanting to be on his own – he just doesn't want me. If I go to nurse him, he just doesn't want it and then he's at it – 'I don't like you' . . . and I'm missing it . . . I miss it more from him because he's very close to me, you know, losing two before him [one miscarriage, one baby died at $2\frac{1}{2}$ months]. I think upon him as me baby, but he just doesn't want to know.

The last two statements hardly seem to go together. In the second interview Connie described herself as warm, saying 'Well you've got to do, haven't you', but in describing her relationship with Carl, said that she was rather cool, the only mother to do so. In a different setting, on a taxi ride with Carl, Connie complained to the interviewer when Carl tried to snuggle up to her, saying that she couldn't bear him being creepy in that way.

Elsie and Eddie
In her reply to the previous question, Elsie complained about Eddie's 'clingy' behaviour and how he wanted 'loving all the time', and it appeared that Eddie was another child who wanted more affection from his mother than he actually got. When asked if they showed affection freely to each other, Elsie said 'Yes', but this does not appear to be the case on her part, as observations in the Family Centre bore out.

Katherine and Kevin
Katherine complained that Kevin did not show as much affection to her as she would have liked, but she seemed to expect him to initiate things:

Not really, no. I kiss him at night time or I say to him . . . I was feeling a bit 'cos he's got a bit offhand. I might turn round and say to him 'You've not given me a kiss today. Go on, give me a love, sit on me knee and give me a love', and then he does. But if I don't ask him, he wouldn't bother.

Katherine and Keith
Katherine's comments indicated that Keith, in contrast to his brother, wanted more affection than he was receiving. She said 'He shows it. He keeps saying he loves me and I'm his friend and everything, you know.' For Katherine, it was Keith that initiated the cuddles.

STRATEGIES OF PUNISHMENT AND CONTROL

When considering how parents attempt to control their children and what punishments they use, it is important to be aware of the aims of disciplining children and the kinds of approaches that can be used. All parents want their children to learn socially accepted behaviours, but differ as to what they expect from the children and what behaviours they will tolerate. Ideally such expectations should take into account what one can reasonably expect from, say, a 3-year-old child. Parents also differ in the type of control and punishment they use to encourage their childen to behave as they would wish. Some parents favour what could be described as a high-profile, rather authoritarian approach to discipline. They – as the adult – are in charge: they intervene in children's squabbles to 'lay down the law', they expect children to obey adults rather along the lines of 'because I (the adult) tell you (the child) so', they favour the use of physical punishment. Other parents prefer a low-profile approach, which emphasises reasoning with the child. They explain why they expect a child to do a particular thing and will use concessions and rewards to bargain with a child. For the low-profile parent, rules are not what adults lay down to children but rather apply to both adults and children and can be open to negotiation. As a result, they are prepared to allow a child some autonomy in decision-making and will not always insist on the child obeying them, but instead will recognise that the child's own activities are of value and a valid reason for saying 'no'. The two approaches are not mutually exclusive but rather at either end of a continuum. A high-profile parent may use a low-profile approach on occasion and vice versa. In the long term, however, if the goal of discipline is for a child to understand why he or she should behave in a certain way instead of just doing so when in fear of physical punishment, then the low-profile approach will be the more effective. Ways of tackling the areas of control and punishment of children with abusing parents are discussed in Chapter 13.

We were interested to see what kinds of approaches these mothers used in disciplining their children. Questions 94 to 117 on the interview schedule asked about causes of disagreement, obedience, the strategies that the mothers used to control their children, and about the use of physical discipline. The mothers were asked what they would do in specific situations, if, for example, the child was busy and the mother wanted something done immediately. The mothers' replies are summarised in Tables 10.1 to 10.5 and a fuller account of each interview is presented below. On the whole, the replies would seem to indicate that the mothers favoured a high-profile approach.

Susan and Sally
Susan expected instant obedience from Sally although she conceded that she rarely got it. Sometimes Susan would then resort to physical punishment: 'If

Table 10.1. *Causes of disagreement between parent and child*

Susan and Sally	Sally shouting at her and demanding attention
Katherine and Kevin	Quarrelling, fighting with Keith. Reminding her of her husband
Katherine and Keith	Whining
Elsie and Eddie	Eddie demanding things all the time
Winnie and William	Gets on Winnie's nerves, especially when he is irritable
Connie and Carl	Nothing in particular
Connie and Colin	Whingeing
Andrea and Alan	Alan answering back and causing friction with his father
Jenny and James	Arguments over where he can go to play. Asking to borrow a pound
Natalie and Nonny	Getting up at 5 or 6 a.m. Getting under Natalie's feet. Jumping on the bed. Making a mess in bed
Liz and Lindy	Tantrums. Controlling mother. Preventing mother from having contact with friends

Table 10.2. *Mother's attitudes to the child's 'busyness' during play, obedience and degree of coercion used by mother*

	Respect for child's busyness	Does child obey quickly?	Mother's reaction to refusal
Susan and Sally	No	No	Spanking
Katherine and Kevin	Some	No	Slaps or sends to room
Katherine and Keith	Some	No	Makes him
Elsie and Eddie	Yes	No	Taps hand
Winnie and William	No	No	Makes him
Connie and Carl	Doesn't arise	Yes	Shows slipper. Makes him
Connie and Colin	No	Yes	Makes him
Andrea and Alan	Yes	No	Withdraws ice-cream
Jenny and James	No	No	Makes him
Natalie and Nonny	No	No	Shouts, threatens
Liz and Lindy	No	No	Makes her

she don't do it at first I just spank her'. She did sometimes try to bargain with Sally though: 'Well you won't get what you're supposed to be getting'. Susan would also sometimes promise Sally a reward in advance of being good.

Susan had used a lot of physical punishment in the past but had gradually come to realise that it was not having any effect:

Table 10.3. *Mother's use of bargaining and control by depriving the child of something*

	Do you ever:		
	Promise a reward in advance for being good?	Say cannot have sweets, TV, etc.	Send to bed/room?
Susan and Sally	Yes	Yes	Yes
Katherine and Kevin	No	Yes	Yes
Katherine and Keith	No	Yes	Yes
Elsie and Eddie	No	Yes	Yes
Winnie and William	No	Yes	Yes
Connie and Carl	No	Yes	No
Connie and Colin	Yes	Yes	Yes
Andrea and Alan	Yes	Yes	Yes
Jenny and James	Yes	Yes	Yes
Natalie and Nonny	No	No	No
Liz and Lindy	No	No	No

Table 10.4. *Mother's use of physical punishment*

	Believes it is necessary to smack	Believes smacking does child good	Smacks in anger	Smacks as punishment
Susan and Sally	No	No	No	Yes
Katherine and Kevin	Yes	No	Yes	Yes
Katherine and Keith	Yes	No	Yes	Yes
Elsie and Eddie	No	No	Yes	Yes
Winnie and William	Yes	No	No	Yes
Connie and Carl	No	No	No	Yes
Connie and Colin	No	No	Yes	No
Andrea and Alan	Yes	No	Yes	No
Jenny and James	Yes	No	Yes	Yes
Natalie and Nonny	Yes	No	Yes	Yes
Liz and Lindy	No	No	Yes	Yes

I don't smack her too much. I don't know, I was spanking her a lot there you know. She really was swearing for ages and I used to spank her at first and then after a bit I stopped it. You see, she seemed to be doing it all the more ... And now she doesn't do it as much because I just ignored it after a bit.

Her replies to other questions indicated that she did still smack Sally but fairly infrequently and that she resorted to other means of punishment such as

Table 10.5. *Mother's use of emotional punishment: withdraws affection, threatens to send child away, threatens with another person*

	Withdraws affection	Threatens to send child away	Threatens with another person
Susan and Sally	Yes	Yes	Yes
Katherine and Kevin	No	Yes	No
Katherine and Keith	No	No	Hospital (for touching genitals)
Elsie and Eddie	No	No	No
Winnie and William	No	No	No
Connie and Carl	No	No	Father
Connie and Colin	No	No	Father
Andrea and Alan	No	No	Father
Jenny and James	No	No	Policeman
Natalie and Nonny	No	Yes	No
Liz and Lindy	Yes	Yes	Yes

depriving her of sweets and television and putting her in her bedroom, rather than 'shouting and bawling at her', which had proved ineffective in the past.

Susan and her husband also used emotional punishment and seemed unaware of how their behaviour could be having an effect on Sally. Susan complained of Sally always following her around and 'shouting after her', demanding attention, saying this was the main cause of disagreements between them. From observations of Sally in the Family Centre it appeared that she was an emotionally insecure, attention-seeking child. It hardly seemed surprising, knowing that Susan often told Sally that she would not love her anymore if she behaved like that, threatened to send Sally away and threatened her with an imaginary person 'outside the window'.

Well we had a wee baby up at our house . . . and we say to her, her dad says to her, 'If you don't start behaving, you know, I'm going to get this baby, you know. You can go there.' She screamed all the murder. Jealous as heck she was. 'I promise I'll be good', she says.

Katherine and Kevin

Katherine's reply to the question on causes of disagreements between her and Kevin revealed her concern about her husband's epilepsy and how it might affect her children – a concern she had not voiced before despite her long attendance at the Family Centre:

Just this quarrelling and that, fighting and that – that's all really. Sometimes he um, he reminds me of his dad – sometimes things that he does. I mean his dad still lives with us like, you know, but he's, he's epileptic his dad and sometimes I still have it in me mind sometimes that they might be like him, you know, and that. And it's daft really because he's not like him – it's in my mind I think, most of the time. Even Keith's more like his dad now to me – the way he walks and his ways. And I says to him [her husband], I've spoken to him you know, and I've said 'I'm not having it', and I try my best you know, to do everything for those kids you know, to make sure they do grow up normal. 'Cos he's not normal, John. He doesn't really you see, 'cos half his brain's gone. The fits he's been having – I mean he's not all there. He's not mental, he's working and everything, but he's forgetful and he doesn't remember things and he doesn't remember what we've done and this and that you know, that gets on me nerves you know – I don't like it. I don't want them to grow up like that. I have to keep them active – their brains active you know.

Katherine would sometimes respect the validity of Kevin's busyness, particularly if she asked him to do something which on reflection she thought she should probably be doing herself. She was not prepared to bargain with him though, and would not offer him a reward in advance for being good. If she asked him to do something he really had to do, she found she had to keep on at him to do it. If he still refused:

He gets a slap you know, if he keeps going on that he's not going to do it. I slap him for it – or he goes in the bedroom.

Katherine believed it was necessary to smack children but she seemed to smack fairly infrequently, although she was prepared to say that she did sometimes smack when she was angry or depressed. When asked whether she believed in smacking she replied:

Yes I do. But like I said most of the time – I mean at one time I used to think – but the Matron doesn't agree with me, smacking children. But I think now and again they need a smack, but most of the time they go into their bedroom and they don't like that. They come out in about half an hour or an hour, depending on how bad they've been, and it seems to calm them down. But sometimes off hand they get a slap you know, and it's quick, it's all over with.

Generally Katherine did not use emotional punishment but she admitted that she had threatened to send Kevin away on occasions and she seemed to be aware that she should not have done so:

I did do once – at one stage I did – a few weeks ago – and I was thinking to myself, you shouldn't say things like that. No, I don't agree with that, no.

Katherine and Keith

Katherine was one of the few mothers who considered both sides of the question on the causes of disagreements between herself and Keith – although without much success.

I don't know what I get on his nerves, but I know that he gets on my nerves with whining all the time . . . Even when I've smacked him he still carries on. In the end I put him in the bedroom.

Katherine had already answered this interview schedule with regard to her elder son, Kevin, some time previously. Even so, this mother seemed to volunteer a great deal of information. If Keith was busy with something and Katherine wanted him to do something else, her attitude was uncompromising. This reply was in relation to tidying up:

If he said no, I'd make him do it . . . When I've got hold of him to drag him to where he was playing to move his toys, he's got them up. He's never rebelled against me.

Obedience under these circumstances is not altogether surprising. Katherine said, however, that she usually had to 'go on' at Keith to get him to tidy up. If something absolutely had to be done, Katherine again showed a high-profile style:

I'd get hold of the thing and push it into his hand.

Katherine did not promise rewards. She also said that she was not keen on smacking, preferring to withdraw sweets. Katherine thought that smacking tended to make her children worse, not better. If sent to his bedroom, Keith would play with his toys, 'so I don't win with him'. Katherine was, she said, at that time trying to work out a form of punishment that didn't involve smacking. She tended to give in if she had refused him sweets, and give him some anyway when his brother was having them. She would not tell him that she did not love him, and had only once threatened him with an external authority figure. He would not own up to something unless found out. Katherine exerted some pressure to apologise.

In the course of this part of the interview, Katherine remembered that she found it effective as a punishment to take away a toy that Keith was enjoying playing with. She played down physical punishment. On another question, however, concerning arguments with other children, she related two incidents, one at the Family Centre and one at home, when Keith had thrown a toy at another child:

They tell me downstairs [in the Family Centre] that it was like temper with him – he didn't actually mean to throw it at the child but the child was in the way . . . if he'd been at home I'd have given him a good hiding . . . I belt him for it because I know it's dangerous.

Elsie and Eddie
Elsie said the main cause of disagreements between herself and Eddie was Eddie 'demanding things all the time'. Eddie generally did not do as he was told and Elsie veered between two opposite methods of dealing with it:

Just try to ignore it, but sometimes I do get a bit mad.

Elsie appeared to respect Eddie's busyness, saying she would leave him to it if he said he was playing, but one wonders whether this would always be the case given her other comments. She complained that Eddie would not do as he was told and if he really had to do something she 'taps him on the hand'.

Elsie had definite views on what a child should or should not do, not being prepared to bargain with Eddie:

I think that's wrong – giving them what they want just to do a thing for me.

When confronted with her child's actual behaviour, she seemed at a loss as to how to cope with it. She did not think smacking 'works':

No, you know all the time I've smacked him and smacked him, he still won't do it.

She would try and ignore Eddie's behaviour but conceded that often she would smack him, particularly if she was in a bad mood, and be almost unable to stop:

If I'm in a bad mood he has to sort of stay out of me way 'cos he knows I'll sort of lash out at him and I won't stop. Just leave it, but sometimes I can't. Sometimes I smack him and I do go a bit far sometimes.

Elsie did try to use other strategies such as depriving Eddie of sweets or sending him to his room rather than smacking him, although she found the latter strategy not particularly effective. However, it seemed likely that Elsie's lack of consistency was the real culprit. Some of the time Eddie could do exactly as he liked and his mother would ignore him no matter how hard he tried to provoke a reaction. At other times, Elsie would suddenly and immediately lash out at him.

Winnie and William

When asked about causes of disagreement, Winnie said that William got on her nerves when he was irritable. Winnie would like William to obey her straight away, but showed some knowledge of her own child here:

He's the sort of kid what blocks himself off – he only wants to hear when he wants . . . otherwise he don't want to know.

Winnie found she had to keep repeating herself until William did as he was told. She did not respect the validity of William's own busyness:

Make him do it. I don't bully him. I just say 'Come on William.'

Winnie did not bargain with William or promise him a reward in advance for being good, but she did deprive him of things he liked, such as ice-cream or television, if he was naughty. Also William was quite often sent to bed, which he did not like. It transpired elsewhere in the interview that William could not open his bedroom door from the inside, so he was effectively shut in his room. Winnie tended to do this rather than use physical punishment, and although she did smack William, she only did so infrequently and for specific things rather than in anger:

Well sometimes you have to smack them when they're really naughty, like swearing – things like that. But I don't really – the only time I smack him is when he swears.

Winnie was quite adamant that she would not use emotional punishment. She would not say that she would not love William if he was naughty or threaten to send him away:

No, 'cos then he'll think you hate [him] – he hates you then. No, I don't do that.

Connie and Carl

Connie was the only mother who could not think of a cause of disagreement between herself and her child:

I can't answer that one because it doesn't really get on top of me – because Carl on the whole he's good.

However, she also said in reply to another question that Carl never wanted to do as he was told and that she expected him to obedient. If he was not, she made him:

Well, like, if I say pick something up and he won't, I just pick him up and bend him down to pick it up.

Connie's replies on physical punishment also contained ambivalences:

No, I'm right against smacking. I've only ever done it once and I've regretted it you know. But as far as I'm concerned now, the slipper's enough – just showing that and they'll behave.

When asked whether the slipper had ever been used, she replied:

Once, you know, to make them understand that it could be used, and they've never actually disobeyed me since.

Other replies indicated both that she did sometimes smack Carl and also the effectiveness of the slipper:

I've only got to show a slipper and he'll do as he's told.

The underlying impression was that the slipper had in fact been used on more than one occasion.

It also appeared that when Carl attempted to follow behaviour guidelines, he could find that rules would change suddenly:

The other day he got hold of the jampot all over me kitchen – he came and told me. I smacked his leg for it. He said 'You smacked me' I says ' I know, look what you done.' But he told me you know.

Connie did not bargain with Carl; she would not promise him a reward in advance for being good. She would deprive him of sweets and also tell him that she would not take him to the park. She did not send him to bed or stop him watching television. She would not withdraw affection or threaten to send him away, but she did threaten him with his father – although she claimed it was ineffectual:

Just his father – but it doesn't work. Does it heck. He plays him up worse then me, he does. He don't look up to his dad – does he heck – his dad's one big laugh.

Connie was interviewed again a year later, and her responses may well reflect the fact that she was being interviewed for a second time. If she asked Carl to do something and he said that he was busy, she said that she would give him time, or that Colin would do it. She said that she had to keep on at him to do things, but that she rarely smacked him. She would promise him sweets for being good. Returning to the question of smacking, she said that she would have to be very angry to smack, as she knew that it was dangerous. She would not stop him watching television as a punishment: 'he learns from it'. She would send him out of the room into the hallway. She would not tell him that she did not love him, or that she would send him away. This account has some consistency with her account of Colin; in both interviews, she said that she rarely smacked them.

Connie and Colin

Connie was very clear on the aspect of Colin's behaviour that annoyed her:

His whingeing. All the time. If he's not out playing, he's inside, whingeing. He drives me up the wall.

Generally, Connie thought that Colin was obedient:

But if he goes too far I'll smack him. I just can't stand him sometimes. I've got a load of patience but the whingeing – it gets anybody.

If Colin was busy when Connie wanted him to do something, immediate obedience was expected. He would generally obey quickly. He would often be offered a reward in advance for being good. As regards frequency of smacking, Connie said that she smacked infrequently, between once a fortnight and once a month, and then only in anger. She thought that smacking only made children act up 'all the more' and that it was better to 'find something that they like and then not let them have it'. She would also put them to bed if they were naughty. Sweets would be withdrawn as punishment. She would not, however, tell Colin that she did not love him. The only threats that she would make concerned her husband: 'with his dad. But it only made them worse, you know.' Colin would not own up to having done something naughty before he was found out. If he denied having done something, Connie would 'turn round to him and say what a liar you are'. Connie did not exert any pressure to apologise.

Andrea and Alan

For Andrea, the only source of disagreement was Alan's answering back. Andrea saw this as a problem as her husband would smack Alan for this:

His dad'll go to smack him and then I'll sort of grab Alan and say 'He's only a baby.'

Most of the time, Andrea said, Alan did not want to do as he was told. Andrea was one of the few mothers who said that she would give Alan time to finish something off before doing something that he had been asked to do; however, this did have its drawbacks for Alan:

If it's a little thing I've asked him to do, I'd just do it myself . . . then I'll say 'Well don't ask me for sweets later on, because I won't give you any.'

Alan would not generally obey quickly, and Andrea would threaten withdrawal of his afternoon ice-cream as punishment. She would also promise sweets as a reward.

Asked whether she considered smacking necessary, Andrea said that she had

smacked him myself, but not to an extent where you've got to use all your force. Not that kind of smack. I have sort of smacked his hand.

It did appear, however, that her husband smacked the children rather more often:

I always say, well one in a family is enough for all the smacking and shouting and that.

Andrea gave the impression that her smacking was comparatively gentle, 'not to the certain extent where, you know, he's screaming in pain'. Whether Alan's father was administering this kind of punishment is another question.

Andrea would only smack when angry, and said that after leaving Alan alone for a while she would then make friends with him again. This might tend to indicate a more personal style of parenting than that of some of the other mothers. She would use threats – for example, sending him to bed – but 'he'd make more mess if I sent him upstairs'. She had occasionally gone as far as starting to undress him, but said he had never got as far as the bedroom. She would not say that she would not love him, or threaten to send him away. Andrea had used her husband as an external figure of authority:

I used to frighten the children a lot if they were naughty . . . I used to say 'Wait 'til your dad comes home.'

When asked why she had stopped threatening the children with their father in this way, she replied:

Because they were frightened of their dad at one time. There's only Alan that has the guts to stick up for himself, you know.

Alan would own up if he had broken something, but would try to blame someone else. Andrea valued apology only if Alan really meant it. Again, this was a sensitivity to the child as a person that was not seen among the other mothers.

Jenny and James

It was an unusual behaviour that Jenny complained of in James: he frequently asked her to lend him a pound! They also tended to argue about where he could go when playing out. James often tended not to do as he was told. Jenny demanded obedience:

He knows when I shout I mean business. I don't even have to hit him any more. I didn't get anywhere by smacking him anyway. But he knows when I'm angry. He'll say 'I'm sorry mam.' He'll do it then.

Jenny also poked fun at the interview schedule. When asked what she would do if she had asked James to do something for her and he had said 'No, I can't do it, I'm busy', she replied:

Well, after I'd finished laughing, I'd make him do it.

Jenny said that James was generally fairly quick to obey, as 'he always knows how to take me'.

James would be promised sweets sometimes as a reward for being good, but in general Jenny felt that this was a bad idea, as he would come to expect them every time. She said that she rarely smacked him:

I've not smacked him for ages, now, but I think, now and then, they do need a smack, you know, when they've got used to you shouting.

Jenny appeared to avoid smacking. On one occasion when she had been shouting at James he had crept under the bedclothes and she had left him alone and gone to take a Valium. In general, she felt that smacking was not particularly effective, although she had tended to smack him far more when he was younger:

I used to just snap . . . I'd just snap and hit him. I never thought, like you plan, 'I'm going to hit him' . . . I don't even think I'm going to hit him, I'll just do it. Whereas that time I did hold myself back, whereas before it was just a case of crack and that was it, I didn't even know I was going to do it myself.

With regard to other means of control, Jenny said that she would occasionally threaten to send him to bed, but his tears were enough to make her stop:

He's crying then so that's enough.

Jenny would not say that she did not love him because she knew that that would frighten him. She did, however, threaten him with policemen, saying that the police would take him away if he was naughty:

I always threaten him with a policeman and he's scared to death. I don't know if I'm doing right or wrong by doing it but he is frightened of a policeman . . . It's better than hitting them, isn't it?

Natalie and Nonny

Natalie was able to give a long list of things that caused disagreements between Nonny and herself. These included getting up at 5 or 6 o'clock in the morning, getting under her feet in the kitchen, jumping on newly made beds, and eating jam sandwiches in bed:

She does things like eating jam butties in bed in the morning. I mean, the other morning the social worker came, the social services came, and I had just woke up and I didn't notice or anything on the bed and the woman came in, I looked, and bloody bread and jam butties everywhere. I was so embarrassed, and I said 'Excuse me' – taking bloody jam butties to bed – I said 'You naughty little sod.' But otherwise I don't shout. I do when I'm really down and depressed and things. Everything gets on my nerves then. Not just one thing but everything, and it really rattles me up so I just have to put her on the landing.

Some of Natalie's difficulty seemed to arise out of living in a single room with her child, and the tension that she felt was understandable. She, too, acknowledged this problem.

When asked about Nonny's obedience, Natalie said that this reflected her moods, and that Nonny was sensitive to these. Again, Natalie described this problem in rather florid language:

When she knows that, she'll play on it and she won't do anything I tell. I mean I have to tell her a dozen times. Like on the road, for instance, I was ruddy mad at her. She runs across the road and it gets on my nerves . . . When she's on her own sometimes she drives me up the bleeding wall. She won't do anything I tell her.

When asked what she did about it, Natalie said:

Shout at her. Say 'Bloody do it.' My husband once said 'You shouldn't threaten her all the time. You should do it, not threaten her', because I'd threatened to smack her you see, and he said 'Smack her once and she'll know what she's done', you know, instead of saying I'm going to smack her in a minute. I never hit her you see, but the other day I did. I smacked her and she realised. She didn't cry, she just shut up. So I think I'll do that more often. Instead of warning her once or twice, warn her once, and if she doesn't do it, smack her on the legs . . . As I said to my husband, 'If she doesn't do something and if I had to smack her every time, she's not going to feel it at the end, she's just not going to take any notice', so after telling her all the time I think it's better if I did that and then give her a good hiding. Then she'll realise that it's harder than smacking, you know. She a right, you know, a little swine.

It was obvious that Natalie felt that smacking could be a good means of control. Asked what she would do if Nonny did not leave something that she was doing when asked, Natalie again showed her high-profile approach to discipline. If Nonny did not obey she said that she would shout at her, and, if that were not effective,

pull her away from what she was doing and get her to do what I want her to do.

If Nonny refused to do something that she really had to do, she would be smacked. Nonny was never promised rewards for being good.

Returning to the question of smacking, Natalie again showed that she smacked quite often, despite her earlier comment that she had not smacked Nonny often:

. . . three or four times a day, but other days you don't have to smack her at all.

Natalie said that on days when she was in a bad mood she was more likely to smack. She tended to smack when angry, rather than as a planned punishment. She did not withdraw privileges, such as sweets or television, and did not send Nonny to bed, thinking that bed should be for sleeping, and that sleep should not be seen as a punishment.

A question on love withdrawal produced a particularly telling response. When asked whether she ever told Nonny that she wouldn't love her if she behaved in a certain way, Natalie answered:

No, but I have told her that I'll give her away sometimes . . . I mean, 'If you don't behave yourself I'll give you away to your dad', or 'I'm going to put you away where there's lots of other children, and I don't want you'. But I've never said I don't love her. I always say after a few minutes, 'Well, you know Mummy and Daddy really love you, so stop messing about.' But I never say I don't love her.

It is quite likely that these kinds of comments might be very hurtful to the child. Further, it was entirely believable that Nonny really was spoken to in this way: on one occasion Natalie told the interviewer, in Nonny's hearing, that she was planning to send Nonny away to her relatives overseas. It does not appear to have occurred to Natalie that this kind of discipline might be very distressing for the child.

Natalie commented that Nonny would often admit to having done something wrong before she was found out. Natalie exerted considerable pressure, it appears, to make Nonny apologise.

Liz and Lindy
As a cause of disagreements, Liz mentioned Lindy's tantrums. She said that Lindy was generally obedient, and that her means of controlling her varied, depending on the situation: sometimes punishment, sometimes concessions and sometimes bargaining. If Lindy was busy, however, and something needed to be done, Liz would insist on immediate obedience, although Lindy tended to be slow to obey:

I leave it for a while, but in the end we'll get there.

Liz did not offer rewards for Lindy being good:

No, I think when they get to school they'll find that hard.

Discussing the subject of physical discipline of children, Liz said that she used to smack Lindy 'a lot':

My smack, each time, got a little bit harder until I hurt her. That worried me, so I went to Social Services . . . Now, I'll tap her on the hand, I'll smack her on her bottom, but in the past, Lindy's had some pretty bad bruises on her head . . . my first reaction was to lash out. She'd have the knuckle marks and everything on her head . . . all that's stopped now.

When asked how she coped with her anger, Liz replied that she'd feel her temper:

just rising a little bit – so I'd give her a smack then that's it. I know I've got to sit down and calm down because my temper, it goes up and up and up and I explode . . . if I exploded too much I could really hurt Lindy. I have to be so careful, and think twice before I do smack her.

In reply to the question 'Do you think smacking does any good?' Liz said:

Honestly, no. If anything, it makes things worse. It's far better if I can sit her on my knee and talk to her very firmly and chastise her . . . but sometimes a little smack is much better than mental cruelty, which I had as a child.

Liz continued:

it depends what kind of mood Lindy's in, 'cos, you know, they're all individuals . . . you can't compare them with another child at all.

When asked whether she ever threatened Lindy with another person, such as a policeman or a teacher, Liz replied that in the past she had said

'If you're a naughty girl I'll send you back to Mrs Goodbody' [whom Lindy had been in care with], which upset her terribly and I didn't realise . . . that I was being cruel to her . . . She's very sensitive. She'd think about that for weeks . . . it would stay in her little mind. It wouldn't move.

CONCLUSIONS

The mothers differed considerably in the extent to which they saw their children as individuals with individual needs. They also differed in their feelings towards the expression of affection between themselves and their children. Some mothers said that they kissed and cuddled a lot, some that they wished that their children were more responsive to their overtures. A couple of mothers seemed indifferent, whilst others appeared actively to discourage cuddling as 'babyish' or 'being creepy'. Some explained a lack of affection in terms of earlier aspects of their relationships with their children – for example Liz, who expressed clearly her difficulty in showing affection as a result of a bad start to her relationship with Lindy.

None of the mothers appeared to have achieved a completely satisfactory approach to the discipline and control of their children. Only five mothers believed it necessary to smack, yet all smacked their children, either in anger or as punishment. It is very striking, though, that none of the mothers thought that smacking their children did any good at all, indicating a difference between what the mothers thought and what they did. Liz identified the escalation of violence described by Patterson (1982) that can arise out of a reliance on physical punishment as a means of control, and several mothers acknowledged its dangerousness. At times when the child's compliance was essential, several of the mothers described the use of physical force in coercing their child into the desired activity. Few of the mothers would bargain with their child, promising a reward in advance for being good, but most would withdraw treats such as sweets and ice-cream. Threatening the child with another person rarely had any effect.

These children were, it should be remembered, attending the Family Centre nursery on a daily basis, where they were disciplined and controlled through a combination of provision of sufficient activities to keep them occupied, praise for good behaviour, bargaining (as the accounts of lunchtimes show) and selective ignoring of unwanted behaviour. Where more strict chastisement was required, 'time out', when the child was made to sit out of activities in the corner of the playroom for a couple of minutes, was used. This was an immediate punishment for very bad behaviour which was very rarely employed. Instances of hostility, aggression and other difficult behaviour were comparatively rare in the nursery.

One key difference between the approaches of the mothers and the nursery staff lay in their point of emphasis. For the mothers, the problem was that of stopping difficult behaviour once it had begun. For the Nursery Officers the stategy was to lessen the probability of difficult behaviour occurring, through the encouragement of constructive alternatives. However, several of the mothers said that they did not believe these measures could work at home and it is possible that the staff were coping too well to be effective models for the mothers. Another difference lay in the variety of alternative methods that the nursery staff could employ – praise, bargaining and ignoring, with 'time out' as a last resort – compared with the tell, shout then smack that seemed to be a well-worn routine for the mothers.

Without going into details of the exact methods of control used by the nursery staff, the following four features appeared to be essential to the successful control of the children in the Family Centre:

1.   An agreed policy that physical chastisement would not be used.
2.   A milieu which emphasised positive and constructive aspects of behaviour, based on a positive view of the child.
3.   Expertise and resourcefulness on the part of the staff, paired with support for one another.
4.   First-hand experience for all staff of the effectiveness of these measures if used consistently.

When the nursery staff's approach is set out in this way, it is perhaps easier to see why the mothers often felt that they could not discipline their children in the same way at home: the staff presented a model of mastery, not coping. Half the mothers thought that physical chastisement was necessary, and of the remainder who did not, most would smack in anger. All smacked their children at times. They tended, as a group, to focus on negative aspects of their children's behaviour, and were often under considerable stress and lacking in the resources and support necessary to provide a positive environment filled with constructive alternative activities for the child. Finally, because of the structure of the Family Centre, few mothers watched their children with the staff in the playroom, and therefore missed the valuable experience of seeing exactly how these methods could work. A reorganisation of the geography of the Family Centre so that the mothers became more involved in their children's activities might have been helpful. This kind of experience alone could be particularly useful to the mothers, and might help to foster expertise, resourcefulness and a positive attitude, which in turn could lead to a reduction in physical means of chastisement. Hence, rather than trying to change attitudes directly, first-hand experience might be the most useful teacher. Videotaped examples of different approaches could also have been useful, were equipment available.

Is it justifiable to encourage parents to use forms of discipline that may be outside their usual range of experience and which run counter to their own upbringing and background? Possibly it is. A large proportion of these children would not comply with their parents' requests unless under considerable duress, and for many of them physical discipline had spilled over into physical abuse. As Chapter 11 on follow-up shows, some of the children who had been most clearly out of the control of their parents continued to make very poor progress in the long term. For this reason, guidance for parents on alternative forms of discipline may be a very helpful form of intervention.

11   *Follow-up*

One of the main aims of our work was to take a long-term view, and to see the psychological characteristics and development of the children in relation to the kinds of experiences that they had had with their families, and also with peers and other adult caretakers. For this reason, we felt that our study would not be complete without some kind of follow-up of the children with whom we had been so closely concerned, if only for a comparatively short time. The first planned follow-up took place 18 months after our period of data collection at the Family Centre, when the Matron was interviewed in order to obtain information on each of the children and their families.

We had hoped to be able to carry out the same rigorous form of school follow-up as that reported in Chapter 2, two to three years after we had worked with these children. Unfortunately, however, we were not permitted to follow up the children either in school or through the NSPCC once our research grant ended. The reason for refusal given by the local Child Abuse Policy Committee was that it was unethical to collect information on any child without the parents' full and informed consent being given. We did not feel that we were able to renew our relationship with these families after so long a period out of contact with them, and were unable, therefore, to collect any further information beyond the interview data that we had obtained from the Matron of the Family Centre, for which we were extremely grateful.

THE FOLLOW-UP

In the autumn of 1983 the Matron of the Family Centre was approached and asked for any information that she had on each of the children whom we had worked with. This follow-up, made 18 months after we had ceased all research contact with the children, yielded a great deal of information, although we had the feeling that the Matron's perennial positive set towards the children may have flavoured her accounts of their continuing development to a considerable degree.

The amount of information available on each child varied greatly: some of the children had ceased to be active cases some time before, whilst others were still in the thick of family problems. The Matron's comments, gleaned from a

172

wide range of sources, are given below. We include a brief summary of parent and child, based on observations reported earlier, as a preliminary to each report.

Susan and Sally

Susan had described how she and Sally were 'more like sisters' and had liked to 'muck about together'. They had enjoyed doing things together and there were many positive aspects to their relationship. Sally, however, was a very attention-seeking child, with low self-esteem, who liked a lot of individual adult attention. She was insecure and became jealous if her mother took notice of another child. Sally had tantrums, and needed firm control, and could be aggressive to both children and adults. Her mother had little idea of how to control her, or how her own behaviour might affect her child. Although Susan no longer screamed at Sally, she still used emotional punishment which appeared to increase Sally's insecurity.

Susan would continue to need help in laying down clear guidelines for Sally. The marital relationship was poor and Susan received little support from her husband. It looked as though Sally would have problems adjusting to the school setting, and that the time between leaving the Family Centre and starting school would be crucial. The family would need support in settling Sally into school, and it was hoped that the discipline there would help to offset any continued lack of discipline at home.

Follow-up

In the period between Sally's participation in the research project and follow-up, her father had left home. Sally's mother appeared to be unable to cope with her. Sally was being allowed to 'run wild', and was not being sent to school. Away from the support and supervision of the Family Centre, the mother was unable to control her young child. No comment was available on Sally's adjustment to school, but her non-attendance had been reported.

Elsie and Eddie

Elsie was attached to Eddie, but because she was rather withdrawn and of low ability she found it difficult to appreciate her lively and amusing son. He already appeared brighter than his mother. Elsie had no consistent approach to controlling Eddie; she tended to ignore his behaviour completely and let him do as he liked. While his mother watched television, Eddie would run out of the flat and 'play out' for hours – a dangerous practice for a 3-year-old. The only way that Elsie was able to get him to do anything was by physically making him do it, or by physical punishment.

Eddie appeared attached to his mother, although wary of her on occasions.

He would throw tantrums to try and get his own way with her, but no longer did this with the Nursery Officers at the Family Centre. Elsie would need help in developing her parenting capabilities; she needed to learn what was appropriate and inappropriate behaviour for a 3-year-old, and techniques for handling manipulative behaviour. She also needed to be encouraged to be involved in activities with Eddie and to talk to and play with her child.

Follow-up

Reports from home and school showed that Eddie was behaving very differently in the two settings. At school, he was managing well, liked by his teacher as a polite child. At home, he was running rings round his mother, stealing money from her, and presenting her with serious behaviour problems. The Matron identified the root of the problem as being the difference in intelligence between mother and child. Eddie, with his superior intelligence, was highly manipulative with his mother, and their relationship continued to be chaotic. Elsie would characteristically give in to Eddie when conflicts arose, in a kindly manner, not realising the problems that she was creating for herself. Eddie continued, in consequence, to be unaware of any boundaries or rules at home that he should obey, for none were set for him. As the Matron put it, 'If we say no, OK. If mother says no, he goes ape.'

Winnie and William

Winnie was a rather cold, immature, rigid young woman, who was very controlling in her handling of her children. She favoured the use of physical punishment and, although she did not use emotional punishment, she failed to realise that many of William's frustrations and tantrums arose because he was unable to meet her extremely high standards. Winnie generally did not make it clear why she expected him to behave in a particular way.

William did not appear ready for school; his concentration was poor, his language was often unclear and he appeared to live in a world of his own. Winnie was still involved with a violent boyfriend, which meant both she and her children lived in fear of his violence. For William, this also meant long periods locked in his room. Winnie needed to be encouraged to show warmth towards her children and to play with them, as well as to set more realistic standards.

Follow-up

Little change had been seen in William's home circumstances; his mother was still having the same problems with her violent cohabitee. William was one of the only children not thought to have made a good transition to school; he had encountered problems settling in.

Connie, Carl and Colin

Connie was an articulate women, preoccupied with her own problems, who often appeared to have little time for her children. Her descriptions of life at home had included many inconsistencies, and discipline appeared to alternate between lax and harsh approaches. Carl was a bright child, solitary in the playroom, who had at first shown an unnerving habit of rolling his eyes upwards so that only the whites could be seen. He had been described by the staff as 'a real Oliver Twist'. He looked sickly and undernourished, was underweight and showed emotional disturbance. He appeared wary of his mother, and protective of his younger brother Colin, who had suffered injuries. He appeared to attempt to shield his brother from his mother.

Colin was also inclined to seek out a 'safe spot' in the playroom, and watch all that went on around him. The two brothers could sometimes be seen locked in apparently painful physical combat, biting and pinching, which often took place in total silence. Colin was a very likeable, cuddly little boy, but watchful and dependent on his older brother.

Follow-up

Both Carl and Colin were thought to be well settled into school at the time of the follow-up, and were coping well. Carl was thought by his teachers to be a particularly intelligent little boy. Connie was, perhaps, the biggest surprise. She was extremely well liked by their teachers, being seen as a wonderful woman who managed her family very well. She was also developing a reputation for being very good with children.

Katherine, Kevin and Keith

Katherine and Alex had long-standing marital difficulties and Katherine blocked Alex out of the family. In some ways Katherine appeared to care for her children well: they were fed, clean and healthy, and did not show signs of developmental or language delay, although Kevin did wet the bed at night.

However, we had often felt anxious about these children. Their mother's attempts to frighten and upset them, her apparent fascination with their sexuality and Keith's inability to relax were just a few of the aspects of the family that gave us concern. Katherine had swings of mood, and there was a suspicion of a drink problem. Keith was still appearing with occasional cigarette burns, and she was very negative towards him. By the end of the research period he appeared a very unhappy little boy.

Follow-up

The follow-up did not offer much hope for the continuing development of the children. Katherine was said to be the same as ever, and still making extravagant calls for help at the slightest difficulty. She had arrived drunk at school one day to collect the children. Another day she had fainted at school, a behaviour identified as an attention-getting device by NSPCC staff. More seriously, she had cut her wrists in front of Kevin some four to five months before follow-up, knowing that her social worker was on the way to the house.

Keith, who had previously escaped serious injury, had put his foot through a washbasin two months previously, and had had his leg in plaster for some time. Whether this had been an accident or a deliberate injury was not certain. The week of the follow-up the children had again been taken into care. The Matron's feeling was that Katherine's drinking was a central problem, and one that she should be able to overcome if she had sufficient concern for her children. At school, the children were said to be fine, and apparently enjoyed the time spent there.

Liz and Lindy

Liz had suffered periods of depression and anxiety, and had found it hard to establish a warm relationship with Lindy, who had been a low birth weight baby and the product of an unhappy relationship. Liz had talked of her guilt over the many blows that she had dealt Lindy, and of her explosive temper. An incident during which Lindy had been burnt against a gas fire had never been resolved. Liz continued to be emotionally abusive to Lindy in the Family Centre at times, but their relationship appeared to be improving. Liz attributed this to the Family Centre, saying that she now felt much closer to Lindy, and appeared to enjoy her child as a person. They were noteworthy at lunchtimes for their prolonged and friendly interactions at the meal table. Some of Lindy's comments indicated a degree of role-reversal, and protection of her mother.

Lindy had at first appeared inclined to play the victim in the Family Centre, was accident-prone, and given to much crying to attract the attention of staff. At this time she was the only girl in the Centre. With Nonny's arrival, however, she appeared much more content, and the two played long and imaginative games together. Throughout the second period of research she appeared to change from a lonely, hostile and unhappy child to one much more able to make relationships with others, and play appropriately. Throughout, she was inclined to fight when challenged, and could deliver an impressive vocabulary of swear words. Overall, however, mother and child appeared to have made a great deal of progress in the Family Centre.

Follow-up

Lindy's follow-up began sooner than we had intended with distressing surprise. Only days after the end of our research association with her, Liz had made an attempt on Lindy's life. Liz had, it should be remembered, been appearing to make gain after gain in her personal adjustment, in her relationship with Lindy, and in friendships with others. She had been asked out on a date; she saw her increasingly good image of herself confirmed; her life was on the way up. Suddenly, it all went wrong: her date stood her up. Her new confidence destroyed, Liz was again unable to cope. As Lindy slept that night, her mother approached her, carrying a plastic apron, and pressed it down over her child's head, waiting for her to suffocate. Lindy did not. She woke up, struggling and screaming, and fought against Liz, who gave up her attempt and called her social worker.

Lindy went straight into care. The next day, at the Family Centre, Liz was in with her social worker and, seeing her, trembling and distraught, her face white and frozen, it was tragic to remember how well everything had seemed to be going in the preceding period. This mother–child dyad had been, to us as researchers, one where we had felt confident of a good prognosis, but as this incident showed, their existence together was fragile, as though balanced on a knife-edge.

A year and a half later, we found that Lindy's case had been closed. Her mother had gone for psychiatric treatment immediately following the attack on Lindy, and this appeared to have been successful. Lindy began to come home on visits of ever greater duration, Liz did everything that was asked of her, and there were no more problems or traumas. Lindy was said to have made a happy and successful transition to school, which she loved, and where she was thought to be a bright, intelligent little girl. It was felt among the staff in the Family Centre that her experience at the Centre had stood her in good stead for the demands of the school environment.

Natalie and Nonny

Natalie had very high expectations of Nonny, and nagged and scolded her a great deal. Natalie had separated from her husband, and now had a very rapid turnover of boyfriends, one of whom had wanted Nonny to watch their lovemaking sessions. Nonny often had to sit on the landing of the flats where she lived whilst her mother entertained boyfriends in their one-roomed bedsit. Natalie was characterised by hypochondriasis, and was given to telling fabulous tales of her illnesses. She tended to be unpopular with the other mothers.

Nonny appeared a very 'normal' child: animated, bright and lively, friendly and talkative, given to rather explicitly sexual play with James. She took guidance from the Nursery Officers very well, and appeared to have no major problems in adjusting to the nursery setting. Although Nonny had to take second place to her mother's other concerns, Natalie appeared to have some sensitivity to her child's personality and needs.

Follow-up

Nonny was another child who appeared to have reached a happy state of affairs with her mother. They were comfortably housed in a flat that had been the envy of all the other mothers in the Family Centre, and Natalie seemed to have passed through her promiscuous phase while under the umbrella of the Family Centre and to have entered into a period of greater stability and calm. There had been no new emergencies or problems, and the case was now closed. Nonny was doing very well at school, and seemed happy and contented.

Andrea and Alan

Andrea had talked of Alan with great affection, and appeared to have much love and affection to offer her children, whilst being rather inclined to let them 'take over' and run rings round her. Her husband had injured Alan's older brother, and there were fears that Alan too might be injured if he were at home all day, as his father continued to be intolerant of his three children and was inclined to be violent. A major reason for attendance at the Family Centre was respite for Andrea, who needed assistance in learning ways of controlling her children. With the help of the Family Centre, she appeared to be succeeding.

Alan was characterised in the play room by the degree of opposition that he showed to anything that was suggested to him. Once settled to play alone, he would sit quietly for a long time. At large in the playroom, however, he would attack other children both physically and verbally, and he maintained a strong position as 'top dog' with the other children.

Follow-up

Alan's progress continued to be good. He seemed to have no real difficulties. Throughout further problems with her husband, Andrea had maintained a good relationship with Alan, and mother and son gave each other a great deal of pleasure. The Matron felt that the Family Centre had provided a useful separation for Alan and Andrea, allowing Alan to escape from his mother's desire to 'baby' him. Alan was said to have settled well at school.

Jenny and James

Jenny had talked of James with great affection, and appeared to appreciate his playfulness and sense of humour. However, she was cohabiting, on and off, with a violent man who frequently drank to excess and was intolerant of James, and James had suffered a great deal of disruption and unhappiness as a result. James's behaviour at the Family Centre deteriorated throughout the period of observation. He was clearly very anxious, and probably depressed, and these emotions expressed themselves behaviourally in the form of tantrums and aggression alternating with periods of helpless sobbing and inertia, during which the staff cuddled and comforted him. His mother talked of his many fears, including a recurrent fear that she might die and leave him alone. James clearly needed kind, firm handling, and consistency and continuity of relationships in order to allow him to feel more secure.

Follow-up

Little information was available on James's progress. James was still living at home, and Jenny had just had another baby. Her cohabitee appeared to be coping rather better. At school, James was apparently making satisfactory progress.

CONCLUSIONS

The follow-up showed very considerable differences in the kinds of experiences that the individual children had had, and the quality of the adjustment that each child had made to his or her home circumstances. What was sad to observe was the extent to which the psychological environment in which some of the children were living appeared to be substantially unchanged. Hence William, Kevin and Keith, Eddie and Sally appeared still to be living in families which were failing to provide an adequately warm and consistent environment. More optimistically, however, the majority of the children were reported to have made a satisfactory transition to school, and the Matron's opinion was that their Family Centre experience had prepared them well for the constraints and demands of the school environment.

In a follow-up study of 6-year-old children who had attended the Family Centre some years previously, Gregory & Beveridge (1984) found significantly higher levels of maladjustment when these children were compared with non-abused peers, using the Bristol Social Adjustment Guide. Their findings of higher levels of over-reaction for the abused children is in accordance with the results of the study reported in Chapter 2. Measures of school attainment, for example vocabulary and arithmetic, showed no significant differences. This would tend to indicate the value of using a range of tools for assessment in examining the long-term effects of abuse.

Unfortunately this option was not open to us. The refusal of the Child Abuse Policy Committee to allow us to follow up the children in school was made from a clear moral and ethical standpoint, and, perhaps appropriately for 1984, was concerned solely with the protection of confidentiality of information surrounding the families that we had worked with. The decision does, however, raise broader ethical issues concerning research in this area. These are largely outside the scope of this book, but we would suggest that some research cannot be done with the full and informed consent of all concerned, and that, in such a sensitive area as child maltreatment, it is necessary to temper one's approach to one's subjects with the constant knowledge that what may seem an innocuous research procedure to the researcher concerned may be extremely threatening to a parent, and hence potentially dangerous for the child. For this reason, we approached our work with the families on the overt basis that we were primarily interested in the children. This was true, but we were also very interested in the mothers.

We stand by the Newcastle follow-up as morally justified, even though the parents of the children concerned were not informed. We feel that the procedures used were adequate to ensure confidentiality of information, and further, that the data collected were of value in highlighting the continuing poor development of children who were supposedly no longer in need of specialised professional attention. Such data in the present study would have enabled us to tie down with some precision some aspects of early experience that might predict poor adjustment to school, and, by reflection, to highlight areas of early mother–child interaction that might merit intensive therapy. The discussion in the next chapter goes some way towards exploring these kinds of variables.

12   *Child abuse: ways forward*

As the earlier chapters of this book have shown, concentration on physical injury in legislation concerning maltreated children and intervention with abusing families can lead to a great deal of important information on family functioning and on psychological aspects of the child's development being missed. Chapter 2 showed that despite intervention with families in which non-accidental injuries (NAI) had occurred, a substantial proportion of the children concerned appeared maladjusted when compared with their peers at school. As the descriptions of the children in the Family Centre have illustrated, physical injury *per se* formed only a small part of the maltreatment to which they were subjected.

In Chapter 1 we discussed the ways in which problems of definition contributed to this state of affairs. If, as we suspect, emotional abuse and emotional neglect play by far the most significant role in the poor development of these children, then two major issues are raised. The first of these concerns the way in which child maltreatment is to be conceptualised in future, and the second, leading from this, is the way that the services should be organised in order to provide the best possible care for children at risk of maltreatment of any kind. Society needs to move beyond the restrictions of legal definitions towards the provision of care tailored to the best interests of the individual child – a concentration not just on pathology but on constructive ways of enhancing development for children who have already suffered major setbacks. To fulfil this aim, research that addresses these issues needs to be carried out and its findings utilised.

THE RELATIONSHIP BETWEEN RESEARCH AND PRACTICE

The nature of current research is such that most studies of child abuse tend to produce averages and summaries derived from comparisons of large groups of abused and non-abused children. This kind of work has produced important findings, which have led to the development of theory, and further research aimed at a better understanding of child maltreatment. Indeed, child abuse has been one of the major 'boom' areas of research in the USA in the last decade.

Unfortunately, this large-scale approach tends to be of comparatively little help in practice, where the 'average abused child' does not exist and each child and family requires an approach that is tailored to their particular characteristics and needs. Research can, of course, offer important pointers to areas that are likely to be problematic, and may suggest areas for resource development at a planning level. Research can also offer a conceptual framework within which to work. However, the majority of research in child abuse is probably inadequate for guiding the day-to-day work of therapy with individual families.

Gelles (1982), after spending 10 years carrying out research into family violence, took for a year a clinical position involving therapy with abusing families. He subsequently wrote:

Perhaps the biggest surprise and disappointment of my clinical experience was how little of the actual research and theory on family violence I actually drew on . . .

(p. 16)

. . . It was sobering to find that after only a few months of clinical work I would find myself forgetting or ignoring the results of my research as I struggled with the emotions, complexities and responsibilities of conducting clinical diagnosis and doing therapy.   (p. 18)

Gelles concluded that some conceptual frameworks could transfer well between research and therapy and that there were benefits to be derived from a research background. Major differences, however, lay in the distinction between the individual approach and the experimental or statistical approach to a problem. The therapist would aim to include the circumstances and events that were unique to the individual and work with these over time within a unique therapeutic alliance. The researcher, on the other hand, would look for a comparatively narrow set of dimensions or factors along which groups of individuals might be expected to vary, and, over a short time span, use efficient standardised measurements in order to make generalisations about the group of interest.

To take a possibly rather extreme example, a study reported by McCabe in 1984 produced evidence derived from physiognomic measurements that the cranial and facial characteristics of abused children tended to appear older than those of carefully matched non-abused controls. This study would appear to be of theoretical importance, as the findings might explain why certain children tend to be singled out for abuse: their physical characteristics lead parents to have unrealistically high expectations of the developmental level they should have attained. It therefore links biological with social and psychological explanations of abuse. The result is, however, of very little immediate value to the individual practitioner; most probably the research will be ignored. This is a pity, as the findings could suggest to a practitioner dealing with a rather mature-looking abused child that it would be useful to ask the parents in rather more detail than usual about age-related expectations; the indentification of these could be an aid to therapy. The finding could also explain why one particular child in the family is singled out for abuse. For therapeutic purposes, however, the research is of largely academic interest. At best, it acts only as a weak pointer for the practitioner at the assessment stage, and is unlikely to have any impact on the therapeutic procedures used. What practitioners need is research directly relevant to their immediate problems, that suggests simple, direct ways of making assessments and indicates likely areas of successful intervention.

How can research be made useful to practice? Some of the best literature ought to arise from research carried out by practitioners with their client groups. For many reasons, however, the majority of therapy remains a private experience between therapist and family. Even the most highly motivated practitioner finds research difficult; generally there is simply insufficient time for it, and research is viewed as a luxury, saved up for the day when the waiting list is less pressing.

A second, related issue militating against research during therapy is the commitment that the practitioner has to maintaining the best possible therapeutic relationship with each individual client or family. The use of standardised measurement procedures may seem to run counter to this. Research traditionally requires restraint and restriction of behaviour on the behalf of the experimenter, in order to avoid bias or skew of results. Hence, we were unable to play with the children in the Family Centre for considerable periods of time when engaged in formal observation, and restricted our discussions with the mothers to the format of the structured interview, rather than dealing with the issues that the mothers themselves might have wanted to raise.

In practice, the special relationship between the client and professional is necessary; influencing the client towards change is at the heart of the therapeutic process. There is, therefore, a tension between the requirements of the two roles of therapist and researcher. One possible solution to this fundamental problem may lie in an individual case study approach.

THE CASE STUDY APPROACH: A NEW PARADIGM FOR APPLIED RESEARCH?

A useful change of emphasis in research could come in the form of a swing away from large-scale, extensive and rather superficial studies towards a body of case studies based on reports of individual therapy cases. There is considerable support for such a change from a number of sources. Using this approach the practitioner, guided by a clear hypothesis, would take a number of measures of functioning or behaviour at the initial assessment stage and repeat these at intervals during therapy, while at the same time documenting the nature of the intervention, the course of therapy, and probable reasons for changes seen in the child or family over time.

To take an example, a social worker interested in the impact of therapy on child behaviour could make standardised observations of some specific aspect of the behaviour of an abused child in a nursery setting at intervals throughout a period of intervention, and later relate these to stages in therapy with the family. This would provide the social worker with a measure of the child's functioning, and familial variables appearing to exert an influence on this. A study such as this would arguably be of more value to a practitioner faced with a family presenting similar problems than would a large-scale study of many families with a less practically based focus; it would augment the knowledge already available from colleagues who had faced similar difficulties in therapy.

The development of a body of detailed case studies offers not only considerable potential for improvements in therapeutic procedures, but also potential for theoretical growth. A body of such studies allows the identification of common themes or strands between cases, and the specification of a greater number of factors likely to be involved in child maltreatment than those that might be seen in a larger-scale study.

TOPOGRAPHICAL DESCRIPTION VERSUS FUNCTIONAL ANALYSIS

It is comparatively easy to draw parallels between families on the basis of their common topography: family size, composition, income level and so forth. Many studies have considered the contribution of these kinds of variables to abuse. Others have considered, for example, general psychological characteristics of the parents likely to contribute to abuse. Such studies provide a valuable overview of variables likely to be of importance. The kinds of conclusions that they can reach are, however, limited; the backgrounds and characteristics of many abusing parents – for example a history of family discord, social isolation, poverty and so on – are actually characteristic of a considerable percentage of the population.

The question that remains is why specific children in specific families become subject to abuse. One step towards answering this question would be to work out a formulation of the kinds of psychological features and processes that characterise the individual family. Such a formulation would be unique to that family, and be based on detailed assessment. Further, where maltreatment of the child appears to be a continuing process, as in the case of several of the families described in this book, it is important to see what function, if any, is served by the maltreatment.

To take an example from the child abuse literature, scapegoating of a particular child is commonly mentioned as a cause of maltreatment. One could ask, therefore, what function this process fulfils for the family. While the simple labelling of a familial process as scapegoating can be termed a topographical description, one can proceed towards an analysis of the function of the scapegoating within the family, that is, from a topographical description to a functional analysis. Functional analysis as it is described here is derived from the literature on behaviour therapy; Smith (1984) suggests that it should be a first step in planning interventions in abusing families. Owens & Ashcroft (1982) give a useful example of its use in clinical practice.

This kind of analysis allows further consideration of the role of physical and emotional violence within the family. For some of the families described here, violence was not an end in itself; rather it was the outcome of attempts to discipline the child. Physical abuse was the result of a family system in which physical chastisement served the function of maintaining the parents' authority. Jenny injured James by hitting him – a habitual method of control; but as he was standing on a table, from which he fell, his injuries were more serious than might otherwise have been the case. Hitting him had the function of control; abuse was a by-product.

In some families, problem drinking or alcoholism was a central issue, and abuse followed on, again as a by-product. James had suffered his worst injuries at the hands of his mother's alcoholic cohabitee. For such children, functional analysis of the family system would show this dependency as the source of many of the difficulties. Understanding and confronting the function of alcoholism for the dependent individual in the family context might be expected to lessen the probability of future maltreatment. As Smith (1984) has suggested, it may be valuable to look at the affect that accompanies an abusive act, rather than simply the nature and extent of injury.

In a small number of families, where the mothers were borderline psychiatric cases, physical or emotional violence appeared in a rather different context. Liz had a psychiatric history, and her worst attacks on Lindy had come at times when she was least emotionally stable. It was during a period of depression and anxiety that she had first injured Lindy, and acknowledged her own dangerousness by asking for professional help. Her attempt to kill Lindy also came at a time when she was depressed. These attacks served an immediate function in attempting to remove Lindy from her life, and whilst Lindy did not die, she was taken into care for a time. Lindy was also a reminder of past and present failures and so her removal served the purpose of distancing Liz from this source of unhappiness. When Liz was less depressed she did not need to keep this distance from Lindy, and became better able to be warm towards her.

For Katherine, emotional maltreatment of her children appeared to give her pleasure, in addition to enhancing her ability to control them. She enjoyed seeing their unhappiness and fear when confronted with puppets, for example. This emotional cruelty was accompanied by occasional physical cruelty, in the form of cigarette burns and worse injuries, and was perhaps the most long-standing and pervasive maltreatment that we saw in these families. Indeed, it could be argued that where maltreatment rather than harsh chastisement was serving a function within the family, the child might run the greatest risk of physical and emotional abuse.

A distinction could therefore be drawn between abuse which itself fulfils some function, as in Katherine's case, and abuse which is a by-product of other factors within the family, as appeared to be the case with Jenny and James. This distinction could provide an important focus for decision-making and offer clear therapeutic goals. A very different intervention would be suggested according to whether abuse has a functional role or whether it occurs as a result of poor control strategies. Clearly, families do not fall into exclusive categories; abuse may fulfil a different function for different parents within the same family, or a different function for the same parent at different times. Where abuse has multiple functions it could be hypothesised that the child is then at greatest risk of continuous or near-continuous physical and emotional abuse. A single attack on a child can, however, produce severe damage, and it is therefore important in intervention always to work out the antecedents of physical violence and the consequences for the parent.

Formulation of the problem

Using Katherine and Jenny as examples, let us look closely at a possible formulation of the processes in each family. Figs. 12.1 and 12.2 show some of the variables likely to be important in each case. They contain some of the basic information discussed at length elsewhere in the book. The figures are not intended to be definitive statements about each family, but instead highlight particular aspects of the family that might indicate directions for further assessment and therapy. They are open systems of description, amenable to change in the light of any new information. Formulations such as these do not presuppose any one therapeutic orientation, rather they set out the kind of hunches and hypotheses about the family which could guide further assessment and intervention.

Fig. 12.1 shows for Katherine, Kevin and Keith and their family the individual attributes of the family that contributed to their particular way of interacting. The formulation sets out a constellation of problems, including the marital situation and the presence of Katherine's brother in the household, sharing a bed with Kevin. The mother's fascination with her sons' sexuality, her enjoyment of making them frightened and unhappy, and her use of physical punishment are included, as are the emotional outcomes for Kevin and Keith. The main problem for the family appears to be the absence of clear boundaries between adults and children; Katherine behaves like a cruel and inquisitive child towards her sons.

In contrast, Fig. 12.2, the formulation for Jenny and James, shows a relatively narrow range of issues and a rather more straightforward situation. Jenny is tolerant of physical violence as a means of control, but at the same time fails to provide adequate protection for James from her cohabitee.

Both families share topographical similarities in the shape of poor housing,

Fig. 12.1. Diagrammatic formulation of some of the major factors contributing to the current problems experienced by Katherine, Kevin and Keith.

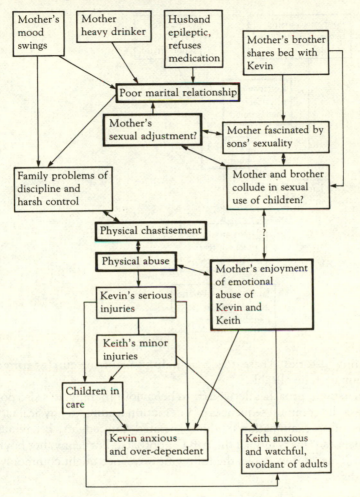

poor relationship between mother and husband or cohabitee, and a reliance on physical chastisement. The formulations suggest very different areas for intervention, however.

Setting out like this the relevant factors in each family enables potential areas for assessment and intervention to be seen. Further, it allows child maltreatment to be viewed as a part of a family system, and highlights the reasons why it is more likely to exist in this family than any other poor family with a history of emotional disturbance. A further piece of information that should be included in the formulation is the contribution made by the parents'

Fig. 12.2. Diagrammatic formulation of some of the major factors contributing to the current problems experienced by Jenny and James.

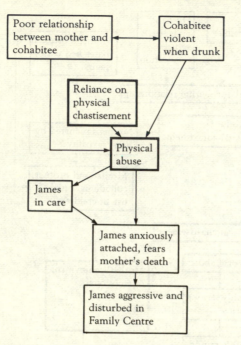

own family histories. These, too, may help to make the current patterns of behaviour more explicable.

Again using approaches derived from behaviour therapy, it is also possible to express the common sequences of interaction leading to physical violence in terms of an examination of the associated antecedents, behaviour and consequences. This is termed the A-B-C approach. For Jenny, her boyfriend Bob and James, for example, the following sequence might commonly have occurred:

Antecedents   Bob drunk, James playing noisely
Behaviour   Bob hits James
Consequences   James is quiet, Jenny runs to fuss him. James's
               bruises are noticed at the Family Centre

When an incident is expressed in this way, it is possible to see that a comparatively simple sequence of activity can be used as a foundation for further conjecture, information-gathering and intervention. For Bob, the immediate outcome of his behaviour is that James stops playing. One intervention would be to encourage Bob either to control his drinking or to move out, using court procedures if necessary to ensure this. Another might be to help him to tolerate James's play. An alternative hypothesis might be that James provokes the scene in order that Jenny will fuss over him. For Katherine, sexual excitement may be one consequence of her abuse of her children. In providing help, one approach would be to take several instances of a family problem – for example, over-harsh physical chastisement – and see the common patterns between incidents. It is important to identify the natural end of the cycle, in order to see why such patterns are maintained.

So far we have spoken primarily of physical abuse, but emotional and sexual abuse can also be included in this model of maltreatment. It is conceivable that in some families over-harsh verbal control of children spills over into abuse, whilst for other families emotional maltreatment has some functional role, perhaps in reliably evoking a particular emotion in a family member. Arguably, sexual abuse is most frequently of the second kind; it is not a direct means of controlling the child, but rather serves some other function in the family.

ASSESSING VULNERABILITY

It is often said that all of us have the potential to maltreat our children but that most of us do not. In Chapter 1 some characteristics of families who abuse children were discussed. Within the scope of functional and A-B-C analysis there is the potential to identify more clearly why specific families are particularly at risk of child maltreatment. It is important to consider the family's previous history and experiences, current pressures and strains, and beliefs about child rearing. The parent who is already inclined towards harsh physical control may physically injure; the parent disposed towards verbal control may emotionally abuse. Martin & Walters (1982) discuss the extent to which different forms of abuse arise in different families.

The specific family's susceptibility will be influenced by personal experience and history at all levels – from society, neighbourhood ecology and social relationships through to individual psychological variables. The work of Garbarino & Sherman (1980) on neighbourhood variation in rates of abuse is a good example of one aspect of susceptibility; McCabe's research on facial and cranial characteristics is another, from the other end of the spectrum (McCabe, 1984). A careful description of the individual family, based on a functional analysis, allows the contributions of these variables to be seen; the origins of a specific vulnerability are clearly central to therapy. Meddin (1985) goes some way towards providing specific criteria for assesment of risk.

CONCLUSION

Within the scope of the approaches presented in this chapter there is the potential for the development of a general model of abuse. The potential is there to collect a large number of observations from expert practitioners with a common ground in therapy. The potential is also there to identify more clearly the variables that contribute to abuse in specific families, to see common vulnerabilities, to examine instances of abuse in ways that may allow help to be optimally directed, and to assess the relative value of different therapeutic procedures. Ultimately, it is practitioners who are most likely to undertake the kinds of studies that are most relevant to their immediate needs. This chapter has attempted to provide some pointers towards this goal.

13 Putting the child first: some practical issues

As we have seen in the preceding chapters, abusing families present with many different problems, and the children may express the effects of their experiences in disturbed and difficult behaviour. Many of the children followed up in Chapter 2 were showing aggressive, hostile and overtly deviant behaviour, as were some of the Family Centre children, while others were quiet, withdrawn, or prone to watchful behaviour. In the children we studied severity of injury was not the major determinant of the degree of disturbances that they showed; the family environment that they were continuing to experience was likely to play a far more significant part.

We argued in Chapter 1 that the way in which child abuse is managed depends upon the definitions in use, and it would appear that although current limited definitions of child abuse go a long way towards ensuring the physical safety of the child, these may blind professionals to a wider range of problems experienced by family members, and to continuing rejection and neglect of the child. For therapeutic purposes a broader definition of abuse would be more helpful, and this must be based on a set of expectations on the behalf of professionals that the child is in an environment in which certain needs are being met. As we have shown, it cannot be assumed that the provision of a safe daytime environment for the child and support for the mother is enough to ensure that the child will develop appropriately. We have demonstrated that observation of the child may yield a great deal of information which can be used therapeutically, particularly if the child can be observed interacting with his or her parents.

In this chapter we consider several areas: firstly, the rights of young children; secondly, the importance of a knowledge of the basics of child development and means of assessing this; thirdly, alternatives to physical punishment; fourthly, forms of substitute care; and then, to set these points in context, we look at the case of Jasmine Beckford, whose recent death at her parents' hands illustrates many of the points that we have tried to stress throughout the book. We then consider the multidisciplinary unit as a possible alternative model for the care of children at risk. Finally we look at the way in which social policy follows such an influential case as that of Jasmine Beckford.

191

THE RIGHTS OF THE CHILD

Kellmer Pringle (1974) outlines four basic needs of children: (1) the need for love and security, (2) the need for new experiences, (3) the need for praise and recognition, and (4) the need for responsibility. Here, we set out seven very basic rights, some of which overlap with Kellmer Pringle's. Our aim in doing so is to point out essential rights of the child, and to set these in the context of problems experienced by the families we worked with. These rights are: to be fed, to be clean, to play, to be safe, to be secure, to be valued, and to be allowed to be a child.

1. The right to be fed

People working with young children need to be aware that an underweight, unhealthy-looking child may be in danger. A child may be receiving an inadequate diet as a result of lack of money, or parental ignorance of nutrition. A parent may be withholding food inappropriately as a punishment, or may expect a child to feed him or herself when he or she is unable to do so. Mealtimes may be a source of tension between parent and child.

2. The right to be clean

It requires constant effort to keep young children completely clean; whilst mothers vary greatly in their tolerance of grubbiness, certain basic standards need to be met. The child whose nappy is not changed for days is not receiving an adequate standard of care. A mother may see a dirty nappy as a sign of naughtiness, or may not want to be bothered changing the child. Professionals need to ensure that parents have the basic materials and resources to keep their children clean. A parent who sees a dirtied nappy as a deliberate act of provocation needs help.

3. The right to play

Play is the 'work' of the child. From the beginning, children need to be talked to, picked up and encouraged to explore their environment. Children cannot develop without stimulation, and at first, adult caretakers are their most important source of stimulation. It is not enough to give children toys and expect them to play with them. A child can develop without toys – indeed, playthings can be improvised from many household items – but a child cannot develop without social interaction. An example of this is Eddie, who did not know his own name because his mother never spoke to him. Professionals need a knowledge of the norms of child development so that they can recognise children who are not developing at an appropriate rate. Certainly, there are differences between children, but most children develop within certain broad parameters: for example, one would expect a 3-year-old to be talking. A child who sits passively in a corner during a home visit by a professional, not making any sounds and not seeking any attention from his or her parents, should not necessarily be perceived as a 'good' or happy child. Children have the right to grow and develop appropriately, and this entails a degree of mess and noise.

4. *The right to be safe*

Children need to be kept safe in a physical sense, protected from dangers in the environment that they cannot yet understand. This involves, for example, parents making their home safe through the use of fireguards, putting dangerous objects, drugs or household chemicals out of the way, and teaching the child about risks, at an appropriate age and in an appropriate way. Katherine 'taught' Kevin 'not to mess with the fire' by holding him against it. This is inappropriate teaching which amounts to abuse. The same is true of burning a young child with matches to teach him or her not to play with them. Similarly, expecting a young child to remember a rule after only one telling is inadequate teaching.

A child should be safe from physical assault. Professionals need to be aware that the use of continual physical punishment can easily deteriorate into habitual physical abuse. They must respond clearly on this issue and be able to present workable alternatives to parents (see below).

A child should also be safe from sexual assault. Most sexual abuse of children occurs within the family and until recently its incidence was grossly underestimated. Professional and concerned adults need to be alert to the possibility of sexual abuse. Throughout the book we have stressed the value of observation; no clues that the child's or adult's behaviour may give should be ignored, and children must have the means to seek help (Elliott, 1985). A child who cannot speak about his or her experiences can be helped through the use of dolls and play therapy techniques. Finkelhor (1984) provides an excellent account of the present state of knowledge in the field of sexual abuse.

5. *The right to be secure*

A child should be safe from fear: fear of violence, sexual abuse, or other assaults from others in his or her social world. It must be remembered that where one parent is abusing a child, the other parent is failing to protect that child. A child who lives in fear cannot be free to explore the world without constraint, and thus is blocked in learning and development. An insecure child will be an anxious child and may, as we have seen, show a range of disturbed behaviours. Some of these behaviours, for example hypervigilance, may have adaptive value at home, but the child's development is hindered as a result. A child may be locked into negative behaviour as a means of gaining attention. Often, parents do not provide clear guidelines for good and bad behaviour, or do not adhere to any consistent rules. The child will be confused as a result, and will be unable to respond appropriately. Professionals need to be active in taking the child's behaviour into account and to be aware of the possible sources of different forms of difficult or withdrawn behaviour. They must also be able to observe the child's response to adults, both parents and others, and whether the child's behaviour changes according to whether or not his or her parents are present.

In order to be secure the child must be free from emotional abuse. Such abuse can take many forms, as we have illustrated. Rather than looking for elegant definitions of abuse, professionals need to be aware of the appropriateness or inappropriateness of things that parents say and do to their children, and to observe the child's response. Parents often make idle and confusing threats which may diminish the child's sense of security. If parents frequently tell their children that they do not love them or that they will send them away, or lock them up for hours and ignore their distress, or frighten and tease them excessively, then those children will be insecure. They may not show physical signs of abuse, but damage will still occur. It is probable that some parents may themselves have experienced this kind of rearing, and in order to break the cycle of deprivation across generations (Rutter & Madge, 1976) they need help in understanding how their child develops, and encouragement in responding to his or her emotional needs.

To be secure, children need to know that their needs will be met, and that they will not be neglected. The baby left to cry in the cot or pram for hours without food or comfort will be less secure. Children need to know that someone will care for them not only in terms of routine feeding and changing but also when they are uncomfortable or lonely.

6. The right to be valued

Children need to feel valued and of worth; they need to feel that they are loved, and that they are appreciated for themselves. A child needs encouragement and affection in order to grow. Children who only ever receive negative messages about themselves may show low self-esteem and come to expect or even invite failure and rejection. This may affect later relationships, and ultimately they may seek to have a child who will love and value them and make up for the past. This solution may, however, become a problem when the baby cannot meet the needs of the parent.

7. The right to be allowed to be a child

A parent who has a child in order that he or she may be loved will be disappointed. Children are rewarding in their own ways, but they are also very hard work. The process of child rearing is like a continuous problem-solving exercise: each week seems to bring new issues to tackle. For the parent, meeting these challenges appropriately and successfully gives a tremendous sense of achievement. Where this cannot be attained, the parent may feel rejected or let down, and child rearing becomes a burden.

Immature parents who know little of child development are ill-equipped for the tasks ahead. They may interpret the child's behaviour inappropriately, thinking their baby is doing something 'to get at them', or that, as Connie said, the infant 'has the devil in her'. Parents may have unrealistic expectations of their child, and be unable to recognise age-appropriate behaviour for what it is. They may also feel that all was well until they had the child, and hence that any change for the worse is the child's fault, rather than recognising the changes that they need to make in order to accommodate the new family member. All this will militate against the child's need to develop as his or her individual personality dictates. Through the experience of being accepted and understood for what they are, children in turn learn to accept and understand others.

Parenting requires flexibility, energy and much work, and parents who are under stress may need extra support in order to carry through their role successfully. In the following section we suggest that professionals need good training and knowledge of normal child development. Parents need this too. For parents who are particularly at risk, the provision of education and guidance during pregnancy and the early months of the child's life may be helpful. If it is difficult to screen 'at risk' individuals, perhaps this is an argument for providing the same basic resources for training of all new parents. In particular, the parents' expectations of their infant are worthy of exploration, and parents may need to be told, for example, how to toilet-train a child, and at what age this is appropriate. The provision of this kind of advice by professionals is particularly valuable where the parents are without other sources of support or information due, perhaps, to social isolation. Leach (1977, 1983) provides a great deal of useful basic information that could be used in parent education.

NORMAL DEVELOPMENT AND ITS ASSESSMENT

Having a clear idea of the needs and rights of children and of the stages of normal development is a prerequisite for any professional who is to be confronted with a family where non-accidental injury is suspected. Social work training has tended to focus on working with adults and what they say about their children. Such an approach is inadequate when working with young children, and, although the pre-schooler may be unable to explain how he or she is feeling, the child's behaviour will often offer valuable clues. Workers need to be aware of whether the child is showing disturbed behaviours such as delayed or pseudo-mature development, hyperactivity or withdrawal, hostility or over-anxiety to please. In the case of infants, regular weight checks can indicate the existence of an inadequate environment if growth rate is poor. The child's reactions to the parent and to strangers can be observed, and the extent to which movements are age-appropriate can also be taken into account, for example. There are many excellent short texts which set out the more recent research on infants and pre-schoolers and their parents in a comparatively accessible form; Dunn (1977), Hetherington & Parke (1979) and Stern (1977) are examples of these.

If the professionals working with families of abused children had this kind of knowledge they would be in a better position to assess the development of infants and pre-schoolers in their care. We would also recommend the use of trained observers who can watch the children at play and integrate information from this source with other data available. Observation of peer interaction provided a great deal of information on the children discussed in this book. Watching the child interacting with the parents would also be of great value. The use of other developmental tests by trained professionals is appropriate too; testing infants and pre-schoolers, whatever the tool used, reveals much about the interactive style of the child, and can highlight potential problem areas that may need attention.

A further area of assessment used in the present study that we feel was useful was the interview with the mothers. Given the opportunity to talk about their children within a structure that allowed many different aspects of family life to be covered, but which was not strictly problem-orientated, some mothers showed considerable sensitivity to their child's needs. All the mothers talked about areas of family life that were difficult for them, and in one case discussed a fundamental problem for the family that had not previously come to light. Asking indirect questions sometimes elicited rather less socially desirable answers to sensitive topics such as discipline than did a direct approach.

As noted in Chapter 9, the questions on discipline raised the important issue that while all the mothers smacked their children, not one of the mothers thought that smacking did any good. In the next section we consider the question of physical punishment in abusing families and suggest some alternative forms of discipline.

PHYSICAL PUNISHMENT

It is outside the scope of this book to look in detail at intervention with abusing families. However, as we described the use of physical punishment in some detail with these mothers, and because professionals differ widely in their views on the extent to which different forms of control should be suggested to parents, we feel it is appropriate to examine the issue of physical punishment more closely and suggest some ways of working with parents in this difficult area.

There is little doubt that many cases of child abuse arise from physical chastisement that has become increasingly more harsh. At the same time, physical chastisement is generally condoned as a necessary sanction against children, both at home and in institutional settings (see Gerbner, Ross & Zigler, 1980). It is made possible by the child's small stature and inability to fight back, and is probably maintained by the immediate relief that is experienced by the perpetrator when the child appears, however momentarily, to be under control. Older children are less likely to be struck as they might strike back, or point out that the adult is behaving unkindly or unreasonably, and thus confront the adult, in some way, with his or her actions. One danger of physical chastisement is that violence comes to be seen as a solution, rather than a problem.

On her way home from work, one of our friends was unfortunate enough to run gently into the car in front of her at a roundabout, bending the other person's car bumper slightly and causing major damage to her own vehicle. The man in front jumped out of his car, and, towering over her, began to shout. In response to her apologies he grabbed her by the shoulders and shook her violently. The other drivers, held up by the fracas, looked upset but did nothing. Would he have shaken a man of his own size? One wonders how he treats his wife, or what he might do with a naughty child. Would this kind of behaviour be permissible within the family? Violence is unacceptable, but it does occur, particularly when people are tired or unhappy. We need to move towards systems of control of children that do not have physical attack as their mainstay.

Somehow, one might have more sympathy for the driver had he behaved in the same way to a small boy who had been dragging a nail along his car's paintwork. But as the mothers at the Family Centre all agreed, physical chastisement generally tends to have little effect on the specific behaviour that the parent wishes to change. To take an extreme example, if someone disagrees with you, or if they cannot understand the point that you are trying to make, you have little chance of changing their mind by hitting them. It is more probable that you will make them so upset that they will be unable to think about what you have said for some time. Yet this is the approach that is often used with children. Physical chastisement exists in the context of a clear power differential serving to emphasis the existence of that differential; as such it can be fairly effective. Its educational potential is, however, very limited. It is crucial for professionals working with abusing families to be both clear in their approach to the use of physical punishment and able to explore with parents why it may not be an acceptable or effective way of controlling children.

How do professionals react to evidence of or the disclosure of physical punishment by parents? Initially they often give the impression that physical punishment is acceptable – 'We've all hit our children', 'We've all lashed out when we were at the end of our tether' – thus confusing being supportive of the parents in their distress with condoning their actual behaviour. Parents may get the message that 'It's all right as long as you don't go too far', i.e. 'We don't want to see any marks or bruises.' Some parents have become very adept at covering up evidence of physical assault or keeping the child out of the way until the injuries have healed. One of the authors was once told by a social worker 'I tell them if you're going to use the belt, don't use the buckle end.' In their efforts to be supportive of the parents and to be seen as non-judgemental, professionals sometimes seem to forget that it is a defenceless child who is at the end of this battering. They also assume that the parent is quite happy to be using physical punishment and is merely seeking reassurance about this, when the opposite is often the case. As we have seen, many parents feel unable to control themselves when they use physical punishment: they know they go too far and are not happy about it, but they do not know what else to do.

Professionals need to explore the expectations that parents have of their children. Where these are unrealistic, the child is likely to become a target of abuse, as he or she will be unable to match up to the parents' standards. In such cases it would be appropriate to teach the parents what could not be expected of a 2-, 3-, or 4-year-old. It is necessary, too, to identify times of particular tension when physical chastisement is likely to be used. Mealtimes and bedtimes can be particularly difficult for parents and pre-schoolers. The sequences of behaviour that parent and child enter into at these times need to be broken down and examined, so that the parent can identify the moments when he or she may resort to physical punishment.

In this way, both the professional and the parent become aware of the antecedents, the behaviour itself and the consequences – the A-B-C sequence of behaviour. Parents vary considerably in the extent to which they smack in anger (where the chastisement is a release of parental feelings) or because they see it as a necessary punishment for the child. It is also very important for the practitioner to ensure that the parent who administers the physical chastisement is the one receiving help and support. There is little point in convincing the mother of the value of alternative means of control if her cohabitee is going to continue to beat the child up every time he gets drunk.

One problem for the families with whom we worked was the level of stress that they lived with on a daily basis. If parents are stressed they have less time for methods of control that involve a great deal of resourcefulness, such as distracting the child with an exciting game – although this strategy was used to excellent effect in the Family Centre by the Nursery Officers. Some of the mothers had found rewards and bargaining useful, and had been able to use 'time out' rather than hitting their child. 'Time out', where the child is removed from the situation where the problem behaviour is occurring, can be very effective, and need only be used for a couple of minutes.

Below we offer four rules that may be of use in working out alternatives to physical chastisement with parents who are stressed, and limited in their ability to use strategies that require a great deal of energy. This is not an exhaustive set of possible ways of controlling children; as we said at the end of Chapter 10, the Nursery Officers were masters of this craft, and we outlined there the strategies that they used. The four points listed here could be used as a framework with individual parents to enable them to draw up a programme for their child, focussing on specific problems that arise within the family routine.

1. *Decide what the rules are.* Rules need to be age-appropriate and as simple as possible.

2. *Be consistent.* We found that most of the mothers would give their children mixed messages about rules. Sometimes they would enforce the rules vigorously, and at other times laugh at naughty behaviour. Where there are two parents, both must agree to uphold the same rules with the same degree of consistency.

3. *Praise the child for good behaviour.* In many families where children show behaviour problems, these arise because the child only gains attention by being naughty, and good behaviour is ignored.

4. *Explain what you mean and keep explaining.* It is difficult for young children to remember rules, especially when they are absorbed with something or excited. Parents have to expect to explain the same thing many times before the child internalises the rules. If the parent can respect the child's needs, and acknowledge this, there is some hope that the child will become able to behave in the same way towards the parent.

SUBSTITUTE CARE

One of the major care decisions that has to be made in dealing with a case of child maltreatment is that of whether or not the child should be taken from the natural parents. Exploring his own family background, Minuchin (1984), a family therapist, recalls that when his mother was depressed for a time he was sent to stay with his aunt. This did not in any way constitute fostering, but allowed his mother some respite from her responsibilities, and allowed him to enjoy a happier environment. With the geographically and sometimes emotionally distant family relationships that our mobile age has brought us, it is perhaps true that, as Martin (1976) comments, parenting is more difficult for us all, and especially difficult for a few.

Minuchin suggests an adaptation to this state of affairs in the form of foster families that foster the entire family. In this way the child is not 'taken away', but rather, the family as a whole has another family to whom they can turn at times of crises. A parallel to this ideal might be seen in the 'Home from Home' schemes in existence for handicapped children. These provide a consistent alternative home for children at holiday times or times of special difficulty, and, for the parents of abused children, would give the opportunity to seek an alternative viewpoint or advice when in difficulty, and to see more positive attributes in their child. The benefits for the child are obvious. Ideally, this system could be introduced at the ante-natal stage, if a particularly high-risk family had been identified.

As Minuchin points out, however, this requires a non-punitive attitude, and also a generous spirit on the part of the fostering family. Jealousy between the natural and foster parents could be one major obstacle; yet if both families could see the situation as one in which they have strengths to share for a common good, perhaps it could work, for some families. As Martin says, children belong neither to their parents nor to society but to themselves. For some families ways need to be found of helping them to spread the responsibility of caring for children more widely.

For abusing families, where social isolation is known to be a major factor, a consistent alternative family who would not require court orders and official documents before helping to share in child care could be very valuable. This kind of system might lessen the burden on professionals responsible for the dismal task of separating young children from their parents, and at the same time increase the chances of children being able to enter a protective environment when necessary. It would thus help professionals to put the child first in decision-making. For lower-risk families the 'Dial-a-Granny' scheme currently operating in Adelaide might merit consideration (Barbour, 1983).

JASMINE BECKFORD

On 5 July 1984 Jasmine Beckford, aged $4\frac{1}{2}$ years, died of cerebral contusions and subdural haemorrhage as a result of severe blows to the head. It later became apparent that Jasmine had suffered physical abuse over an extended period. Her stepfather, Morris Beckford, was convicted of manslaughter in March 1985, And her mother, Beverley Lorrington, was sentenced to 18 months' imprisonment for neglect. This killing was one of a series in England which appear to be contributing to policy change regarding child abuse, and as such merits closer attention.

The report of the enquiry chaired by Louis Blom-Cooper, QC, appeared on 2 December 1985, and declared Jasmine's death to have been both a predictable and a preventable homicide. One of the critical factors indentified was the pronouncement by the magistrates, on the basis of inadequate knowledge of Jasmine's home environment, that they hoped she could be reunited with her natural parents. The second was the return of Jasmine to her parents after a period of fostering, without sufficient recognition of the level of risk involved. The report identified several other areas of concern which are directly relevant to the material presented in this book.

The level of training of the social workers was found to be inadequate for work in child protection. As we have said in this chapter, professionals working with child abuse cases need a great deal of knowledge of the way in which children develop in 'normal' families. The inadequacies of generic social work training and service provision were highlighted by the enquiry report. The British Association of Social Workers had, in the week before the report appeared, declared that the child should come first in child abuse cases, and it is hoped that training will be provided towards this end. It is unreasonable to provide inadequate training and insufficiently clear guide-lines for social workers and then blame them for being unprepared for the work demanded of them.

One major issue was that the children in child abuse cases are rarely seen by the professionals involved. If, as we suggest, child care professionals had regularly observed the children either with the parents or at play, they would at the very least have seen a bruise or limp, even if other effects of abuse on behaviour had not been noticed.

Further, the report called for concentration of resources into the 'grey areas' of work with families where something more than supervision but less than long-term removal of the child is needed – very much the kind of client group that was attending the Family Centre. It would appear that provision along the lines of a Family Centre, paired with family therapy approaches and intensive work on parenting skills, could be helpful, perhaps on a short-term problem-orientated basis. Residential care provision for the child within the Family Centre, again on a short-term basis, could also be considered. Attendance at such a facility could be seen as a test of motivation on the behalf of the parents to improve their relationship with their child, and where parents refused to take part it could be argued that the child should not be living at home. The kind of fostering arrangement described by Minuchin would also be beneficial at these times of special difficulty.

One of the main criticisms made by the report was that optimism had been allowed to prevail, even though this was not justified. The report stated:

Overweening optimism took hold as soon as the social workers thought they saw the first signs of improved conduct on the part of Morris Beckford and Beverley Lorrington. The prime focus on the parents was never adjusted – indeed it was sharpened as the months at home on trial appeared to be working. Jasmine became the victim of disfunctioning social work that legislatively demanded otherwise – *the protection of the child and not the pressing needs of its parents.* (italics added)

The case of Jasmine Beckford is a clear example of the dangers of putting the parents, rather than the child, first. In Chapter 1 we discussed the impact of the case of Maria Colwell on the shape of child abuse policy for the next decade or more. The effects of Jasmine Beckford's death may well be as far-reaching in policy terms. One likely outcome will be a return towards specialist work with abusing families; already some social workers in London are refusing to take on child abuse cases unless they are trained to do so. Another outcome may be the establishment of more specialist centres such as the Family Centre that we worked in. It is hard to imagine that Jasmine could have suffered in the same way had she been attending such a facility on a regular basis. In the next section we comment on one model of care that might bear consideration as a basis for care of children at high risk of abuse.

THE MULTIDISCIPLINARY UNIT: A MODEL FOR WORK WITH HIGH-RISK FAMILIES

As the last section suggested, it is probable that the next few years will see changes in policy relating to the care of children at risk of non-accidental injury. One possible model for the care of children particularly at risk and their families is offered by some of the adolescent psychiatric services available at present, an example of which is the Young People's Unit in Macclesfield, Cheshire, Here, an adolescent who has reached a point of particular difficulty can be admitted to the Unit for a short period, generally three to four months. The youngster takes part in both therapeutic and educational activities, and the family are involved in the therapeutic process through regular meetings, family therapy and parent support groups. The period of residential care also offers some respite from immediate pressures of family life. The youngster returns home at weekends, often with some kind of task set, and this time at home is considered to be an important part of the process of change. The short stay in the Unit and the time at home also ensure that the artificial environment of the Unit does not come to replace the real environment of home.

The staff of the Unit is made up of social workers, doctors, nurses, teachers, a psychologist and an art therapist, who are all based in the same premises and work as a multidisciplinary team. In addition to daily meetings of all members of the Unit's community and interdisciplinary decision-making sessions, there is a great deal of informal interchange between the professionals. Specialist skills are immediately available: an examination by a doctor can be arranged on the spot; likewise, the skills of any other professional can be called upon with an ease and immediacy that is only possible because all those concerned are under the same roof. At the same time there is tremendous sharing of skills: for example, social workers, nurses, psychologists and doctors all take part in family therapy sessions. Family work is also extended outside the Unit to include other youngsters and their families for whom admission is not necessary, and to follow up families who have attended the Unit and still have issues to resolve.

It is easy to see how this model could be transferred to work with young children. Nursery staff and health visitors could be included in the team, and parent education could also be provided. The Family Centre that we worked in had some of the elements of the team mentioned above, but decision-making was not multidisciplinary to the same extent. At times the Nursery Officers and social workers held quite different views because they had a different focus to their work. The regular meetings at the Young People's Unit which have a common focus of care and in which the views of all professional groups involved are generally given equal weight, provide a good model for the resolution of these kinds of problems.

At the Young People's Unit the youngsters and their families are expected to bring about some form of change during their stay, and are selected on this basis. Areas for change are clearly set out in a contract which is tailored to the family's specific problems. The contract acts as a central focus for the work of the staff and family, with the expectations of both being clearly spelled out. If the contract is broken the youngster may be discharged from the Unit immediately. This shifts the responsibility for change onto the family, while the staff contract to help the family bring about the desired changes. For children at risk, the family breaking the contract might be a point at which to reconsider with them whether or not they wish to remain together as a family, or whether the long-term interests of the child might be better served by the arrangement of an alternative form of care. Harwicke (1985) examines the effectiveness of multidisciplinary work with child abuse cases carried out in Chicago, and suggests that the approach is valuable, particularly with respect to avoidance of fragmentation or duplication of effort, and follow-up.

Regular assessment is an integral part of the work of the Unit. The referral agency, staff, parents and the youngster all complete questionnaires on which ratings are made of current problems. This procedure is followed prior to admission, at discharge and one month after discharge. This allows some formal assessment to be made of the youngster's progress during therapy, and of the efficacy of the work of the Unit. Each youngster is assessed on a series of checklists of emotional and behavioural adjustment during a three-week assessment period following admission. For young children, observational procedures along the lines of those that we have discussed could be very helpful.

One further aspect of the Unit merits attention: two weeks of the year are set aside for training, during which the youngsters are sent home and staff sit down together to learn new skills and work through problems that may have arisen. Outside speakers with special expertise are also invited for talks and workshops. In this way the staff maintain high standards of care, high expectations of change in their clients, solidarity and a fresh perspective on their work.

We saw in the Family Centre that the work with families imposed a very heavy strain on the staff, and stress-related illness was clear. The way that the staff perceive the families in their care, and handle disappointments when a family fails to cope or when they disagree with a casework decision, is an aspect of organisation that needs careful consideration. Multidisciplinary decision-making and regular meetings at which all staff can put forward their points of view on an equal footing is one way of lessening this burden; clear contracts for change with the family as a whole is another. Further, one of the problems indentified in the case of Jasmine Beckford was an unwillingness on the part of white social workers to intervene inappropriately with a black family. With the type of unit described it would be possible to aim for a multiracial staff. Garbarino & Ebata (1983) consider the issues of ethnic and cultural differences in work with abusing families, as do Gray & Cosgrove (1985).

POLICY CHANGE IN ACTION

The newspapers for the first week of December 1985 made interesting reading. On Monday, 2 December, the *Guardian* carried a report of plans drawn up by the Department of Education for a 20% cut in funding for social work training. On Tuesday the 3rd, following the publication of the Jasmine Beckford report, her name was front page news, with social workers, health visitors, magistrates and schools all blamed. The *Guardian* on Wednesday the 4th carried details of the report, and an article which called for better training for social workers in specialist services for child abuse cases, and for a clearer acknowledgement of the duty of social workers to take professional responsibility for children in their care. A separate article in the same paper carried the news that the Department of Education was revising its plans for social work training; a course at one university that had been under threat of closure had now been reprieved. Clearly, changes in policy had already begun as a result of Jasmine's case. What these changes will lead to remains to be seen, but it is to be hoped that, at last, a clearly stated policy will be that of putting the child first.

14   *Looking forward*

If as a society we are sincere about wanting to tackle child abuse, then we need both more resources and better use of those already in existence. We need more practitioners with specialist training and skills in child development, child care and family work. We need more facilities for working with families, more support for families in the community, and a recognition that work with abusing families is a long-term process which must be matched with long-term finance and planning.

While observing the children that we have written about in this book, we became aware that each had developed a different way of coping with the task of living in an abusing family. The emotional damage suffered by some of the children would be carried with them far into the future. As we have seen here, emotional abuse takes many forms, and it would be hard to imagine definitions or legislation that could encompass some of the forms of cruel treatment that we have discussed in the preceding chapters. As we have said before, practitioners need definitions in order to protect children against the worst excesses of their parents, but a therapeutic stance requires a different perspective. If good definitions of emotional abuse cannot be arrived at, perhaps the emphasis should be on looking for the best ways in which individual families can progress in their care of, and interaction with, their children, and on considering what constitutes appropriate as opposed to inappropriate forms of child rearing.

If work in child abuse needs one focus, it might be the task of overcoming the isolation of all involved. Too often, enquiries following the death of a child indicate that many people knew that the child was at serious risk. We need to overcome the isolation of the child within a distressed family; of parents who may be under many pressures and low in resourcefulness; of neighbours who see but feel unable to report abuse; of professionals who cannot always exchange information as freely as they need to, and who are often expected to work beyond reasonable limits and without adequate training. Even the work with abusing families itself is isolated within a tight set of definitions and criteria. We suggested in the previous chapter that community family fostering arrangements and specialist multidisciplinary approaches might go some way towards relieving this problem, and have argued for broader therapeutic approaches to be available to a wider range of families.

Many of the issues that we have discussed are directly relevant to the task of prevention. Even though child abuse has been a focus of concern for many years, help is still being provided after, rather than before the event. The kinds of statistics collected by the NSPCC (Creighton, 1984) do, however, allow the indentification of risk factors, which should provide arguments for extra resources in certain areas of need. The professionals concerned need to be aware of the antecedents of abuse, and to concentrate on times at which children at risk may be indentified.

To take an example, Main & Goldwyn (1984) observed that the ways in which mothers talk about their own childhood experiences of parenting relate closely to the way in which they interact with their own children. What is important here is that it is not some objective measure of the mother's own childhood that is in question, but the mother's perception of her own experience. If a mother of a young child says that her own childhood was unhappy, and that she feels unsure of her ability to rear her child, she may benefit greatly from extra help.

The health visitor service clearly has a major role here, in early detection of problems in the home. The child's progress in other settings can also be scrutinised; non-attendance at nursery should be taken as a potentially important sign. The use of observational techniques in these settings could be particularly valuable; recent research on mother–infant and mother–child interaction has provided many techniques that transfer well to the applied field of work with families (Kennel, Voos & Klaus, 1976; Hyman, 1980; Fontana & Robison, 1984), and we have discussed in this book observational approaches for use in different settings. Identifying problems at this stage relies upon the professional's ability to insist on seeing a child, rather than listening to a parent's reasons as to why this is not possible. The ability to insist on seeing the child in turn depends upon a change in professional emphasis, so that the child is made more clearly the focus of concern.

Many professionals at present may feel that insistence upon seeing the child when the parent will not give permission would constitute a breach of the rights of the family. We have argued throughout this book that the child's rights to health and an adequate standard of care are paramount. If the parents by themselves cannot provide this care, the professionals must find ways of helping the family to ensure that these standards are met. The role of different professionals in relation to the protection of children requires debate and clarification.

One clearly identifiable antecedent of physical abuse is physical chastisement of children. If physical abuse on a major scale is to be prevented, it is arguable that reliance on this form of punishment needs to be reduced. How often clients referred for professional help with a child-rearing problem say that a good belt never did *them* any harm. At the very least, the educational establishment should set a good example here. Given that the school experience is one of the major influences on the development of a child, it would seem important that a model of other forms of control should be set. Rutter *et al.* (1979) have reported that, irrespective of the official orientation of individual schools to physical punishment, higher rates of *unofficial* physical punishment such as slaps and cuffing tend to be associated with poorer behaviour amongst the pupils. These authors speculated that this form of unofficial punishment might set a model of violence for the pupils. This, and other issues of prevention, are dealt with in various chapters in Gerbner *et al.* (1980).

Similarly, Field (1983), reviewing the literature on the incidence of child abuse in different cultures, concludes that abuse is least likely to occur in cultures where there are clearly established, traditional practices of child rearing, strong cultural pressures for the early socialisation of the child, and where there is consistency of child-rearing and disciplinary practices. In agreement with Rutter, *et al.* it would seem that inconsistency in discipline, including physical chastisement, is likely to lead to an increase in violence. This again is an argument for putting considerable effort into helping parents to develop and maintain clear and consistent rules for their children.

Throughout the book we have looked at the consequences for the child of life in an abusing family. For many of the children that we studied family life was a fragmented, confused and unpredictable experience. Perhaps, in time, professionals will be enabled to help families before abuse occurs, through early identification of families who may be at risk. As always, funding is essential. The tools are available; the next step must be a commitment to use all possible skills not just to patch up the tears, but to help the family to weave a firmer fabric of existence around the child.

Appendix. The interview schedule

A. Background

Child's name:
Date of birth:
Age:
Sex:
Family size and position of child in family:

Mother: Age   Not working/working part time/full time?
1.   You haven't had any miscarriages or stillbirths?
2.   Did you have a job before you had children?
Father: Age   Occupation:
3.   Does he have to be away from home at all, except just during the day?
      Home every night/Up to 2 nights away a week/3+ nights away per week/Normally away/Separation or divorce/Dead/Other
      Shift work? Yes/No   What shifts?
4.   Does any other adult live here, apart from your husband and yourself?
      Yes/No   Details:
5.   Has N ever been separated from you for more than a day or two since s/he was born?
      (Details: age at separation, how long, etc.)

B. Independence

6a.   First of all, I'd like to know something about what sorts of things N can do for her/himself. Does N usually dress her/himself in the morning? Do you give her/him any help with that usually?
      Mother helps a lot/some/none
  b. Does s/he undress her/himself at night?
      Mother helps a lot/some/none
  c. Does N tidy up her/his clothes when s/he's taken them off?
      Mother helps a lot/some/none
  d. When N goes to the toilet, does s/he look after her/himself or do you help her/him?
      Prompt: Does N wipe her/himself, or do you do that for her/him?
      Mother helps a lot/some/none
7.   What do you feel about making a child do things for her/himself at this age? Do you think s/he should be made to do things for her/himself, even if s/he doesn't want to?

208

8.   If 'None' was the answer three or more times:
     Have you taken a lot of trouble to get N to do these things for her/himself?
     Would you like N to be doing more for her/himself at this age?
     Prompt if necessary: Does s/he do as much as you think s/he ought to be doing
     now? Do you think you should be stricter than you are over this, or are you quite
     happy to leave it for the moment?

C. Independence in play

9.   How much do you like her/him to do other things on her/his own? For example,
     does s/he ever go into a shop or to an ice-cream van on her/his own?
     If 'danger' or 'distance' response, prompt: But does s/he ever go into a shop on
     her/his own while you wait outside?
     Yes/No   (Specify)
10. Does s/he ever take messages for you?
     Yes/No
11. What about playing in the house? Does s/he like to play on her/his own?
     Mostly/sometimes/not at all
12. About how long will s/he play by her/himself without wanting your attention?
     Up to half an hour/31–60 min/Longer
13. How often do you have to 'start her/him off' and give her/him periodic attention
     during play?
     Often/Sometimes/Never
14. How often does s/he seek your attention when you're busy with something else?
     Often/Sometimes/Never
15. If s/he keeps wanting you to do things for her/him when you're busy, what do
     you do?
16. Does s/he tend to play near you rather than elsewhere?
     Yes/No
17. Does s/he ever come clinging round your skirts and wanting to be babied a bit?
18. What do you do?
     Or: What would you do if s/he did that at this age?
19. Do you think a child of this age should be able to amuse her/himself most of the
     time, or would you expect to have to spend a lot of time on keeping her/him
     happy? (Explain if necessary on her/his own, i.e. without other children)

D. Aggression in play

20. Does N enjoy playing by her/himself a lot or will s/he only play by her/himself
     when there's absolutely no one else to play with?
     Yes/No
21. Does N play with other children at all?
     Siblings: Often/Sometimes/Never
     Others: Often/Sometimes/Never
22. What contact does N have with other children apart from brothers and sisters or
     the children in the Family Centre?
     A lot/Some/None
23. How good is N at sharing and co-operating with other children?
24. What do you do if there's a disagreement or quarrel?

25.   In general, do you think children should be left to settle their own differences at this age or would you interfere?

26.   Suppose N came running to you complaining of another child?
       What do you do?

27.   Do you ever tell N to hit another child back?
       Yes/No
       If yes: Can you give me an example of when you might do that?
       If no: Is there any situation in which you might do that? Yes/No
       Example in either case:

28.   How close is N to the sibling nearest to her/him in age? How well do they play together? How much time do they spend together?

29.   There seems to be two sorts of quarrelling N might get into: quarrelling with her/his brother/sister and quarrelling with other children. Do you find you act differently in those two situations?
       Yes/No
       Rating for encouragement of aggression in self-defence: General encouragement/special circumstances (not age differences)/Never

30.   Does N ever seem jealous of her/his brother/sister/the other children?

31.   *If yes*: What does s/he do when s/he's feeling jealous?

32.   How do you deal with it?

E. Autonomy in play

33.   Does N make a fuss if you give away something of hers/his to another child?
       Does it often happen that you do this?
       Mother wouldn't do this/Might do this

34.   Suppose you were having a good turn-out and you wanted to throw away some broken bits of toys but s/he wanted to keep them: what would happen then?
       Mother wins/N wins/Compromise

35.   If you've broken something of hers/his by accident and it can't be mended, what do you do about it?
       Restitution/Apology/Concealment/Nothing

36a.   Is there any sort of play you don't allow? For example, do you let her/him make a lot of noise in the house if s/he wants to?
       Yes/No

b.   Do you let her/him jump on her/his bed and use furniture for her/his play – like making a train out of chairs?
       Bed: Yes/No   Chairs: Yes/No   Others:

c.   Do you let her/him make a mess playing with water, paint, earth or flour?
       Yes/No

d.   Does it bother you if s/he gets really dirty while s/he's playing?
       Yes/No
       If yes: What do you do to make her/him keep clean?

37.   When s/he's playing at something, do you ever join in? (i.e. games of mothers and fathers, going for a train-ride, shops, etc.)
       Yes/No   Example:

38.   Has s/he any imaginary people or animals or places that s/he brings into her/his play? (*Explain if necessary*: things s/he talks about or talks to, but which don't exist even in the form of dolls?)
       Yes/No   Details:

39.   How do you react if s/he talks about them to you?
        Sympathetic/Unsympathetic

40.   Does s/he sometimes tell you fanciful things that you know are not true, just for
        the sake of telling them? (Exclude lying to avoid punishment)
        Yes/No   Details:
        What do you do when this happens?

41.   Does s/he play games where s/he pretends to be someone like a teacher or a
        shopkeeper or a daddy?
        Yes/No   Details:

42.   Does s/he have a favourite role? Does s/he alternate between several roles? Does
        s/he only play this sort of game when other children are present?

43.   When s/he's playing by her/himself does s/he often use things pretending
        they're something else (for example chairs for a train)?
        Yes/No   Details:

44.   Does s/he ever play any games with rules like ludo or card games?
        Yes/No

45.   What happens if you ask her/him to do something for you and s/he says s/he
        can't because s/he's busy – in the middle of a game or something?

46.   Does s/he make a fuss when s/he has to stop playing? What do you do when
        she does?
        Yes/No
        If necessary prompt: If it's time for a meal and s/he wants to finish something s/he's
        started, what do you do then?

47.   Is there anything special s/he's afraid of, the way some children are afraid of
        insects or the plughole or things at the bottom of the bed?
        Yes/No   Details:
        If yes: Do you know why s/he is afraid of that? Do you know how it started?

F. Meals

48.   I'd like to know something about N's mealtimes now. Is s/he a good eater or do
        you have trouble about that?
        Good/Varies/Finicky

49a.   Do you have any rules about eating up food?
        Yes/No

b.   Are there any foods that s/he never has just because s/he dislikes them?
        Yes/No

c.   Do you let her/him leave food on her/his plate?
        Yes/No

d.   Do you let her/him decide how much s/he will have of a food that s/he dislikes?
        Yes/No

e.   If s/he really refused to eat something, what would you do? *Prompt all mothers*: If
        s/he didn't like a meal after you'd cooked it, would you make her/him something
        else?   Yes/No

49.   *Rating*: Unlimited pressure to finish/child normally has to eat mother's
        amount/Has to eat amount s/he takes her/himself/May leave a little/No
        pressure/Alternative provided after refusal/Other

50.   Do you mind what order s/he eats things in? For example, does s/he have to eat
        bread and butter before s/he has any cake and that sort of thing?
        Strict order/Some attempt but flexible/Doesn't mind

51. Do you let her/him use a spoon instead of a knife and fork if s/he wants to?
    Prompt if necessary: Would you let her/him if s/he did want to?
    No/Discourages/Allows
52. Do you let her/him use her/his fingers? (*Explain if necessary*: for chips, pieces of meat, cut up vegetables, etc.)
    Never/Discourages/Allows
53. Do you let her/him get up from the table during a meal?
    Often/Sometimes/Never/Special circumstances only
54. Is s/he allowed to bring toys or a book to the table?
    Never/Discourages/Allows
55. Do you have any other rules about mealtimes – not talking or anything like that?
    Yes (specify)/No
56. Do you take a lot of trouble to get her/him to eat nicely and have good table manners or are you leaving it for the moment?
    Much trouble/some training/leaving it
57. In general, would you say you mind whether a child has good table manners or not at this age?
    Yes/No

G. Personal habits

58. Going on from table manners now, what about other sorts of habits? Does N have any little habits that you've noticed?
    Check each:
    Hair twisting or pulling
    Thumb sucking
    Nail biting
    Rocking her/himself
    Dummy (if mentioned only)
    Other?
59. Does s/he play with her/himself at all?   Yes/No
    If no: What would you do if s/he did? Would you mind her/him doing that at this age?
60. Is there anything else you can think of that s/he does as a habit? Anything s/he does when s/he's overtired or worried?
61. Do you try and stop her/him (*prompt each one*) or don't you really mind?
    If yes: How do you stop her/him?

H. Bedtime

62. Now what about bedtime? Can you tell me what time N went to bed last night?
63. Is that her/his usual time?
64. Does s/he have to be in bed by any special time?
    Yes/No
65. *If yes*: If s/he didn't seem tired and wanted to stay up longer, would you let her/him?
    Rating: Rigid/Flexibly rigid/Flexible/No rules
66. Does N sleep in a room of her/his own? Own bed?
    Alone/With another (specify)   Same bed?

67. Could you tell me about a typical bedtime from the time you start getting her/him ready for bed to the time s/he goes to sleep?

68. Does anyone else help with getting her/him ready for bed
Other (specify) often takes full responsibility.Other (specify) often helps/Mother alone

69a. Is there anything s/he takes to bed with her/him, like a teddy or a piece of cloth or a bottle or a dummy or anything like that?

b.   Would s/he make a fuss if s/he couldn't find it one night?

c.   Does it have to be that particular toy?

70. Does s/he ever have a bottle now?
Yes/No
If no: Can you tell me when s/he gave it up for good?

71. Does s/he ever suck her/his dummy nowadays?
Yes/No

72. Is there anything special that you always have to do at bedtime – any little game you always have, or something like that?

73. Once s/he gets into bed, is s/he allowed to get out and play around the bedroom?
Yes/No

74. Does s/he have the light on in her/his room for a while?
No light/Night-light/Indirect/Full light for a short time/Other

75. *If full light*: Is s/he allowed to play with toys or books in bed?
If not full light: Would you allow her/him to have the light on and play with toys or books in bed if s/he wanted to?
Yes/No

76. Does s/he have anything to eat or drink in bed?
Yes/No   Details:
What about sweets?
Yes/No   Details:

77. What happens if s/he gets up and tries to come back into the room where you are? Do you ever let her/him stay if s/he doesn't seem sleepy?
Often/Occasionally/Only in emergency/Never

78. Suppose s/he was hungry about an hour after s/he'd gone to bed? Would you let her/him eat at that time?
Yes/No/Only (specify what)

79. Does s/he usually sleep through the night?
Wakes often/Sometimes/Seldom or never?

80. Do you lift her/him for a potty at all?
Yes/Sometimes/No

81. If s/he does wake up, apart from needing the toilet, what does s/he do? Does s/he cry?
Lies awake quietly/Talks quietly/Calls parents/Cries/Very distressed/Seems frightened/Seems angry/Other?
If at all distressed: What seems to be the matter?

82. What do you do about it?
If not mentioned: What would you do:
If s/he seemed frightened?
If s/he was just feeling chatty?
If s/he wanted to come into your bed?
Would you ever:

Let her/him come into your bed?
Yes/No
Get into bed with her/him (if s/he slept alone)?
Yes/No
Sit with her/him?
Yes/No
Get her/him something to eat in the night?
Yes/No
Record if mentioned spontaneously in this section: Stories told or read/Songs/Prayers with child/Cuddling/Kisses

J. Toilet training

83.   You said that you lift/don't lift her/him for a potty at night. I expect s/he still wets the bed sometimes, doesn't s/he?
Yes/No
If Yes: About how often does it happen?
Most nights/1–3 nights per week/Less than once per week/Almost never

84.   *If any wetting:* What do you do if you find s/he's wet her/his bed?
A. Very concerned/Mildly concerned/Unconcerned
B. Punitive/Reproachful/Rewarding/ Neutral or sympathetic
If no wetting: Did you have any problem getting her/him dry at night? Did you have any special method?
Punishment/Reproach/Rewards/No pressure

85.   What about in the daytime? Does s/he still have accidents sometimes?
Yes/No
If yes: Is it mainly wetting her/his pants or does s/he dirty them?
Wet/Dirty/Both/Neither

86.   What do you do?
If punishment not mentioned: Do you ever punish her/him for wetting or dirtying her/his pants?
Yes/No
A. Very concerned/mildly concerned/Unconcerned
B. Punitive/Reproachful/Rewarding/Neutral or sympathetic

87.   Of course most children go through a stage when they think anything to do with the toilet is very funny. Has N got to that stage yet?
Yes/No

88.   How do you feel about children giggling together over that sort of thing? Would you discourage it or just take no notice?

89.   What about children wanting to go to the toilet together or wanting to look at each other when they're undressed? Would you mind them doing that?

90.   Does N ever see you or her/his daddy undressed?
Sees father: Yes/No
Sees mother: Yes/No
How do you feel about that?

91.   Does s/he know where babies come from yet? (i.e. from mummy's tummy)
If no: Would you tell her/him if s/he wanted to know or do you think s/he's too young?   Yes would tell/No
If no: What would you say if s/he asked you?

K. General discipline

92. I wonder if you could tell me now how you and N get on together? What sort of things do you specially enjoy in her/him?

93. Do you show your affection toward each other quite a lot or are you fairly reserved with one another? (*Prompt if necessary*) Do you think kissing and cuddling should be discouraged at this age?
    Rating: Very warm and demonstrative/Warm/Rather cool/Negative

94. What about disagreements? What sorts of things make you get on each other's nerves?

95. Does N often not want to do what s/he's told and what do you do about it? (discounting dangerous situations)

96. Suppose you asked her/him to do something for you and s/he said 'No, I can't do it now, I'm busy'. What would you do? (excluding mealtimes, going out, etc.)
    If no: What would you do if it did happen?
    Accepts/Accepts with disapproval/Gives time/Enforces immediate obedience

97. Does s/he usually obey you fairly quickly or do you have to keep on at her/him to get her/him to do things?

98. If s/he refuses to do something that s/he really must do, what happens then?

99. Do you ever promise her/him something (in advance) as a reward for being good?
    Yes/No

100. How do you feel about smacking? Do you think it's necessary to smack children?
     Yes/No

101. Do you have to be angry when you smack her/him or do you smack her/him simply as a punishment?

102. Do you think smacking does her/him any good?
     Yes/No   In what way?
     Rating:
     A. Smacks only when calm/Only in anger/Both/Almost never
     B. Believes in smacking/Disapproves in principle

103. Is there anything else you do when s/he's naughty?

104. Do you ever say s/he can't have something s/he likes – sweets or television, or something like that?
     Yes/No

105. Do you ever send her/him to bed?
     Yes/No

106. Do you ever tell her/him you won't love her/him if s/he behaves like that?

107. Do you ever say that you'll send her/him away or that you'll have to go away from her/him if s/he's naughty?
     Yes/No

108. Do you ever try and frighten her/him with somebody else – her/his daddy, a policeman, a teacher, a doctor, someone like that?

109. Suppose s/he says s/he hasn't done something naughty when you know quite well s/he has? What do you do then?

110. Does s/he ever come and tell you s/he's been naughty before you actually find out?
     Yes/No

111. Do you think it's important for her/him to say s/he's sorry when s/he's done something wrong? Do you ever make her/him do that even though s/he doesn't want to?

112. Does s/he ever try to smack you or to hurt you in any way? What do you do? Yes/No
    If no: What would you do if s/he did?

113. What about answering you back and being cheeky, and that sort of thing? Do you allow that?
    What about:
    b. Saying mother is silly
    Allowed/Not allowed
    c. Saying 'shut up'
    Allowed/Not allowed
    d.Shouting at mother
    Allowed/Not allowed
    e. Running away laughing at mother
    Allowed/Not allowed
    f. Saying 'I'm not sorry'
    Allowed/Not allowed
    g. Mimicking
    Allowed/Not allowed
    h. Calling names
    Allowed/Not allowed

114. Does N ever have a real temper tantrum? About how often does it happen?
    Most days/Twice or more a week/Once a week/Rarely/Never
    What sorts of things seem to start it off?

115. How do you deal with it?

116. On the whole are you happy about the way you deal with discipline in general, or do you sometimes find yourself doing things you don't really approve of?

117. Compared with other people, do you think of yourself as being very strict, rather strict, rather easy-going, or very easy-going?
    Very strict/Rather strict/Rather easy-going/Very easy-going

M. Baby-sitting

118. How does N seem if you leave her/him with somebody else (e.g. if you go out)? Does s/he mind you leaving her/him?
    Yes/No

119. *If yes:* What do you do about that?
    If no: Was there a time when s/he minded? Age? What did you do?

120. Do you always tell N when you're leaving her/him or do you find it easier to slip off without her/him knowing?

121. How did s/he react when s/he first started coming to the Family Centre? Did s/he mind you leaving her/him in the playroom or did s/he want to come and sit with you in the mothers' room?
    If yes: What did you do?
    Did s/he mind coming on her/his own on the days when you didn't come in?
    Yes/No
    If yes: What did you do? What about now?

N. Changes in upbringing

122. Would you say you've changed your ideas about bringing up children since you started?

NB: Section L (Father Participation) in University of Nottingham Child Development Research Guided Interview Schedule omitted here. Questions 13, 14, 16, 20, 22, 23, 28, 41, 42, 43, 44, and 45 inserted following Light (1979).

References

Aber, J.L. & Cicchetti, D. (1983). The socio-emotional development of maltreated children: an empirical and theoretical analysis. In *Theory and Research in Behavioural Pediatrics*, ed. H. Fitzgerald, B. Lester & M. Yogman. New York: Plenum Press.

Baher, E., Hyman, C., Jones, C., Jones, R., Kerr, A. & Mitchell, R. (1976). '*At Risk': An account of the Work of the Battered Child Research Department*, NSPCC. London: Routledge.

Barbour, P.J. (1983). Adopt a family – dial a granny. *Child Abuse and Neglect*, **7**, 477–8.

Beezley, P., Martin, H.P. & Kempe, R. (1976). Psychotherapy, in *The Abused Child*, ed. H.P. Martin. Cambridge, Mass.: Ballinger.

Bender, B. (1976). Self-chosen victims: scapegoating behaviour, sequential to battering. *Child Welfare*, **55**, 417–22.

Blager, F. & Martin, H.P. (1976). Speech and language of abused children. In *The Abused Child*, ed. H.P. Martin. Cambridge, Mass.: Ballinger.

Bowlby, J. (1953). *Child Care and the Growth of Love*. Harmondsworth: Penguin.

Briere, J. (1984). The effects of childhood sexual abuse on later psychological functioning: defining a post-sexual-abuse syndrome. Paper presented at the Third National Conference on Sexual Victimisation of Children, Washington, DC.

Brown, G.W., Birley, J.L.T. & Wing, J.K. (1972). Influence of family life on the course of schizophrenic disorders: a replication. *British Journal of Psychiatry*, **121**, 241–58.

Burgess, R. & Conger, R. (1978). Family interaction in abusive, neglectful and normal families. *Child Development*, **49**, 1163–73.

Caffey, J. (1946). Multiple fractures in the long bones of infants suffering from chronic subdural haematoma. *American Journal of Roentgenology, Radium Therapy and Nuclear Medicine*, **56**, 163–73.

Calam, R.M. (1983). The long-term effects of child abuse on school adjustment. Paper presented at the 91st International Convention of the American Psychological Association, Anaheim, California.

Cicchetti, D. & Risley, R. (1981). Developmental perspectives on the etiology, intergenerational transmission and sequelae of child maltreatment. *New Directions for Child Development*, **11**, 31–55.

Connolly, K. & Smith, P.K. (1972). Reactions of preschool children to a strange observer. In *Ethological Studies of Child Behaviour*, ed. N. Blurton Jones. Cambridge University Press.

Creighton, S.J. (1980). *Child Victims of Physical Abuse: A Report of the NSPCC Special Unit Registers, (1976)*. London: NSPCC.

Creighton, S.J. (1984). *Trends in Child Abuse 1977–82: The Fourth Report on the Children Placed on the NSPCC Special Unit Registers*. London: NSPCC.

de Mause, L. (1974). The evolution of childhood. In *The History of Childhood*, ed. L. de Mause. London: Souvenir Press.

Dunn, J. (1977). *Distress and Comfort*. London: Fontana.

Dunn, J. & Kendrick, C. (1980). The arrival of a sibling: changes in interaction between mother and first-born. *Journal of Child Psychology and Psychiatry*, **21**, 119–32.

Dunn, J. & Wooding, C. (1977). Play in the home and its implications for learning. In *The Biology of Play*, ed. B. Tizard & D. Harvey. London: SIMP/Heinemann Modern Books.

Egeland, B., Sroufe, L.A. & Erickson, M. (1983). The developmental consequence of different patterns of maltreatment. *International Journal of Child Abuse and Neglect*, **7**, 459–69.

Elliott, M. (1985). *Preventing Child Sexual Assault: A Practical Guide to Talking with Children*. London: Bedford Square Press, NCVO & Child Assault Prevention Programme.

Elmer, E. (1977a). A follow-up study of traumatised children. *Pediatrics*, **59**, 273–9.

Elmer, E. (1977b). *Fragile Families, Troubled Children*. Pittsburgh: University of Pittsburgh Press.

Elmer, E. & Gregg, G.S. (1967). Developmental characteristics of abused children. *Journal of Pediatrics*, **40**, 596–602.

Field, T. (1983). Child abuse in monkeys and humans: a comparative perspective. In *Child Abuse: The Nonhuman Primate Data*, ed. M. Reite & N.G. Caine. New York: Alan R. Liss Inc.

Finkelhor, D. (1984). *Child Sexual Abuse*. New York: Free Press.

Fontana, V.J. & Robison, E. (1984). Observing child abuse. *Journal of Pediatrics*, **105**, 655–60.

Foucault, M. (1976). La politique de la santé au XVIII siècle. In *Les machines à guérir (aux origines de l'hôpital moderne)*. Paris: Institut de l'Environment. Translated in Foucault (1980).

Foucault, M. (1980). *Power/Knowledge*. Brighton: Harvester Press.

Franchi, C. (1982). A detailed investigation of five abusing mothers and their five preschool children focussing on maternal interactive style and its relationship to the child's ability to relate to others. Unpublished Masters thesis, University of Manchester.

Garbarino, J. & Ebata, A. (1983). The significance of ethnic and cultural differences in child maltreatment. *Journal of Marriage and the Family*, **45**, 733–83

Garbarino, J. & Sherman, D. (1980). High-risk neighbourhoods and high-risk families: the human ecology of child maltreatment. *Child Development*, **51**, 188–98.

Gelles, R.J. (1980). A profile of violence toward children in the United States. In *Child Abuse: An Agenda for Action*, ed. G. Gerbner, C.J. Ross & J. Zigler. Oxford University Press.

Gelles, R.J. (1982). Applying research on family violence to clinical practice. *Journal of Marriage and the Family*, **44**, 9–20.

George, C. & Main, M. (1979). Social interactions of young abused children: approach, avoidance and aggression. *Child Development*, **50**, 306–18.

Gerbner, G., Ross, C.J. & Zigler, E. (1980). *Child Abuse: An Agenda for Action*. Oxford University Press.

Gil, D. (1970). *Violence Against Children*. Cambridge, Mass.: Harvard University Press.

Gottman, J.M. (1979). *Marital Interaction: Experimental Investigations*. New York: Academic Press.

Gray, E. & Cosgrove, J. (1985). Ethnocentric perception of childrearing practices in protective services. *Child Abuse and Neglect*, **9**, 389–96.

Gregory, H.M. (1981). The social and educational adjustment of children who have been subject to non-accidental injury. Unpublished Masters thesis, University of Manchester.

Gregory, H.M. & Beveridge, M.C. (1984). The social and emotional adjustment of abused children. *Child Abuse and Neglect*, **8**, 252–31.

Harwicke, N.J. (1985). How effective is the multidisciplinary approach? A follow-up study. *Child Abuse and Neglect*, **9**, 365–72.

Hetherington, E.M. & Parke, R.D. (1979). *Child Psychology: A Contemporary Viewpoint*. London: McGraw-Hill.

Hughes, M., Carmichael, H., Pinkerton, G. & Tizard, B. (1979). Recording children's conversations at home and at nursery school: a technique and some methodological considerations. *Journal of Child Psychology and Psychiatry*, **20**, 225–32.

Hyman, C. (1980). Families who injure their children. In *Psychological Approaches to Child Abuse*, ed. N. Frude. London: Batsford.

Izard, C. & Schwartz, G. (1986). Theories of emotion, emotional development and affective symptomatology. In *Depression in Young People: Developmental and Clinical Perspectives*, ed. M. Rutter, C. Izard & P. Read. London: Guilford Press.

Jones, C.O. (1980). Children after abuse. In *Psychological Approaches to Child Abuse*, ed. N. Frude. London: Batsford.

Jones, D.N. (1982). *Understanding Child Abuse*. Kent: Hodder and Stoughton.

Kadushin, K.A. & Martin, J.A. (1981). *Child Abuse: An Interactional Event*. New York: Columbia University Press.

Kellmer Pringle, M. (1974). *The Needs of Children*. London: Hutchinson.

Kempe, C.H. (1979). Recent developments in the field of child abuse. *Child Abuse and Neglect*, **3**, ix–xv.

Kempe R.S. & Kempe, C.H. (1978). *Child Abuse*. London: Fontana/Open Books.

Kempe, C.H., Silverman, F., Steele, B., Droegemueller, W. & Silver, H. (1962). The battered child syndrome. *Journal of the American Medical Association*, **181**, 17–24.

Kennel, J., Voos, D. & Klaus, M. (1976). Parent–infant bonding. In *Child Abuse and Neglect*, ed. R.E. Heifer & C.H. Kempe. Cambridge, Mass.: Ballinger.

Kinard, E.M. (1982). Experiencing child abuse: effecs on emotional adjustment. *American Journal of Orthopsychiatry*, **52**, 82–91.

Lamphear, V.S. (1985). The impact of maltreatment on children's psychosocial adjustment: a review of the research. *Child Abuse and Neglect*, **9**, 251–63.

Leach, P. (1977). *Baby and Child: From Birth to Age Five*. Harmondsworth: Penguin.

Leach, P. (1983). *Babyhood*. Harmondsworth: Penguin.

Light, P. (1979). *The Development of Social Sensitivity*. Cambridge University Press.

Lynch, M.A. (1976). The critical path. In *Child Abuse: A Reader and Sourcebook*, ed. C.M. Lee. Milton Keynes: Open University Press.

Lynch, M.A. (1978). The follow-up of abused children: a researcher's nightmare. In *Family Violence: An International and Interdisciplinary Study*, ed. J.M. Eekelar & S.N. Katz. Toronto: Butterworths.

Lynch, M.A. (1985). Child abuse before Kempe: an historical literature review. *Child Abuse and Neglect*, **9**, 7–15.

McCabe, V. (1984). Abstract perceptual information for age-level: a risk factor for maltreatment? *Child Development*, **55**, 267–76.

Main, M. & Goldwyn, R. (1984). Predicting rejection of her infant from mother's representation of her own experience: implications for the abused/abusing intergenerational cycle. *Child Abuse and Neglect*, **8**, 203–17

Malone, C.A. (1966). Safety first: comments on the influence of external danger in the lives of children of disorganised families. *American Journal of Orthopsychiatry*, **36**, 3–12.

Manning, M., Heron, J. & Marshall, T. (1978). Styles of hostility and social interaction at nursery, at school and at home: an extended study of children. In *Aggression and Anti-social Behaviour in Childhood and Adolescence*, Ed. L. Heron & M. Berger. New York: Pergamon Press.

Martin, H.P. (ed.) (1976). *The Abused Child: A Multidisciplinary Approach to Developmental Issues and Treatment*. Cambridge, Mass.: Ballinger.

Martin, H.P. & Beezley, P. (1977). Behavioural observations of abused children. *Developmental Medicine and Child Neurology*, **19**, 373–87.

Martin, H.P., Beezley, P., Conway, E.F. & Kempe, C.H. (1974). The development of abused children. *Advances in Pediatrics*, **21**, 25–73.

Martin, H.P. & Rodeheffer, M. (1976). Learning and intelligence. In *The Abused Child*, ed. H.P. Martin. Cambridge, Mass.: Ballinger.

Martin, M.J. & Walters, J. (1982). Familial correlates of selected types of child abuse and neglect. *Journal of Marriage and the Family*, **44**, 267–76.

Meddin, B.J. (1985). The assessment of risk in child abuse and neglect case investigations. *Child Abuse and Neglect*, **9**, 57–62.

Minuchin, S. (1984). *Family Kaleidoscope*. Cambridge, Mass.: Harvard University Press.

Minuchin, S., Rosman, B.L. & Baker, L. (1980). *Psychosomatic Families: Anorexia Nervosa in Context*. Cambridge, Mass.: Harvard University Press.

Mirandy, J. (1976). Preschool for abused children. In *The Abused Child*, ed. H.P. Martin. Cambridge, Mass.: Ballinger.

Morse, C.W., Sahler, O. & Friedman, S. (1970). At three year follow-up study of abused and neglected children. *American Journal of Diseases of Children*, **120**, 349–446.

Newson, J. & Newson, E. (1963). *Patterns of Infant Care in an Urban Community*. Harmondsworth: Penguin.

Newson, J. & Newson, E. (1968). *Four Years Old in an Urban Community*. London: Allen & Unwin.

Newson, J. & Newson, E. (1976). *Seven Years Old in the Home Environment*. Harmondsworth: Penguin.

OPCS (Office of Population Censuses and Surveys) (1977). *Population Estimates 1975. (revised) 1976 (provisional)*. London: HMSO.

Owens, R.G. & Ashcroft, J.B. (1982). Functional analysis in applied psychology. *British Journal of Clinical Psychology*, **21**, 181–9.

Parke, R.D. & Collmer, C.W. (1975). Child abuse: an interdisciplinary analysis. In *Review of Child Development Research*, vol. 5, ed. E.M. Hetherington. Chicago: University of Chicago Press.

Parton, N. (1979). The natural history of child abuse: a study in social problem definition. *British Journal of Social Work*, **9**, 427-51.

Patterson, G.R. (1982). *Coercive Family Process: A Social Learning Approach*, vol. 3. Eugene, Oregon: Castalia.

Patterson, G.R. & Cobb, J. (1971). A dyadic analysis of problem behaviours. In *Minnesota Symposia on Child Psychology*, vol. 5, ed. J.P. Hill. Minneapolis: University of Minnesota Press.

Radbill, S.X. (1968). A history of child abuse and infanticide. In *The Battered Child*, ed. R.E. Helfer & C.H. Kempe. Chicago: University of Chicago Press.

Richards, M. & Bernal, J. (1972). An observational study of mother–infant interaction. In *Ethological Studies of Child Behaviour*, ed. N. Blurton Jones. Cambridge University Press.

Roberts, J., Lynch, M.A. & Duff, P. (1978). Abused children and their siblings: a teacher's view. *Therapeutic Education*, **6**, 25–31.

Rowe, D. (1978). *The Experience of Depression*. Chichester: Wiley.

Rutter, M & Madge, N. (1976). *Cycles of Deprivation*. London: Heinemann.

Rutter, M., Maughan, B., Mortimore, R. & Ouston, J. (1979). *Fifteen Thousand Hours: Secondary Schools and their Effects on Children*. London: Open Books.

Sandow, S. (1979). Action research and evaluation; can research and practice be successfully combined? *Child Care, Health and Development*, **5**, 211–23.

Smith, J.E. (1984). Non-accidental injury to children. 1. A review of behavioural interventions. *Behaviour Research and Therapy*, **22**, 331–47.

Speight, A.N.P., Bridson, J.M. & Cooper, C.E. (1979). Follow-up cases of child abuse seen at Newcastle General Hospital 1974–5. *Child Abuse and Neglect*, **1**, 99–103.

Spinetta, J.J. & Rigler, D. (1980). The child-abusing parent: a psychological review. In *Traumatic Abuse and Neglect of Children at Home*, ed. G.J. Williams & J. Money. Baltimore & London; John Hopkins University Press.

Steele, B.F. & Pollock, C.B. (1968). A psychiatric study of parents who abuse infants and small children. In *The Battered Child*, ed. R.E.Helfer & C.H. Kempe. Chicago: University of Chicago Press.

Stern, D. (1977). *The First Relationship: Infant and Mother*. London: Fontana.

Stott, D.H. (1974). *The Social Adjustment of Children*, 5th ed. London: Hodder & Stoughton.

Sylva, K., Roy, C. & Painter, M. (1980). *Childwatching at Playgroup and Nursery School*. Oxford Preschool Research Project 2. London: Grant McIntyre.

Toro, P.A. (1982). Developmental effects of child abuse: a review. *Child Abuse and Neglect*, **6**, 423–31.

Vaughn, C. & Leff, J. (1976). The measurement of expressed emotion in the families of psychiatric patients. *British Journal of Social and Clinical Psychology*, **15**, 157–65.

Zigler, E. (1980). Controlling child abuse: do we have the knowledge and/or the will? In *Child Abuse: An Agenda for Action*, ed. G. Gerbner, C. Ross & E. Zigler. Oxford University Press.

Zigler, E. (1983). Understanding child abuse: a dilemma for policy development. In *Children, Families and Government: Perspectives on American Social Policy*, ed. E.F. Zigler, S.L. Kagan and E. Klugman. Cambridge University Press.

Reports

Annual Statistical Summary of Cases Registered with the Newcastle Special Unit from Tyne and Wear Metropolitan County and Northumberland (1975). Newcastle Special Unit, NSPCC.

Annual Statistical Summary of Cases Registered with the Newcastle Special Unit from

Tyne and Wear Metropolitan County and Northumberland (1976). Newcastle Special Unit, NSPCC.

A Child in Trust: The Report of the Panel of Inquiry into the Circumstances Surrounding the Death of Jasmine Beckford (1985). London Borough of Brent.

Index